CBIC EXAM BOOK 2019-2020

CBIC Study Guide and Test Prep Manual with Practice Questions for the Certification Board of Infection Control and Epidemiology Exam

Copyright © 2018 by Trivium Test Prep

Certification Board of Infection Control and Epidemiology, Inc. was not involved in the creation or production of this product, is not in any way affiliated with Trivium Test Prep, and does not sponsor or endorse this product.

ALL RIGHTS RESERVED. By purchase of this book, you have been licensed one copy for personal use only. No part of this work may be reproduced, redistributed, or used in any form or by any means without prior written permission of the publisher and copyright owner. Questions regarding permissions or copyrighting may be sent to support@triviumtestprep.com.

CBIC Essential Test Tips DVD from Trivium Test Prep!

Dear Customer,

Thank you for purchasing from Trivium Test Prep! We're honored to help you prepare for your CBIC.

To show our appreciation, we're offering a **FREE *CBIC Essential Test Tips* DVD by Trivium Test Prep**. Our DVD includes 35 test preparation strategies that will make you successful on the CBIC. All we ask is that you email us your feedback and describe your experience with our product. Amazing, awful, or just so-so: we want to hear what you have to say!

To receive your **FREE *CBIC Essential Test Tips* DVD**, please email us at 5star@triviumtestprep.com. Include "Free 5 Star" in the subject line and the following information in your email:

1. The title of the product you purchased.
2. Your rating from 1 – 5 (with 5 being the best).
3. Your feedback about the product, including how our materials helped you meet your goals and ways in which we can improve our products.
4. Your full name and shipping address so we can send your FREE *CBIC Essential Test Tips* DVD.

If you have any questions or concerns please feel free to contact us directly at 5star@triviumtestprep.com. Thank you!

- Trivium Test Prep Team

TABLE OF CONTENTS

About Trivium Test Prep and How to Use this Guide - 5

Introduction - - - - - - - 7

IDENTIFYING INFECTIOUS DISEASES

Terminology- - - - - - - - 13
How Infections Work - - - - - - 23
Causative Agents - - - - - - - 25
Reservoirs and Transmission - - - - - 37
Occurrence, Incubation and Communicability - - 47
Diagnostic and Laboratory Tests - - - - 53
Epidemiology - - - - - - - 57
Antimicrobials - - - - - - 63
Environmental Monitoring - - - - - 67

SURVEILLANCE, ANALYSIS AND CHANGE

Surveillance - - - - - - - 69
Research and Data - - - - - - 79
Rates - - - - - - - - - 107
Risk - - - - - - - - - 113
Quality - - - - - - - - 117
Implementing Change - - - - - - 123
Outbreaks and Breaches - - - - - 131

PREVENTING AND CONTROLLING TRANSMISSION

CDC Guidelines - - - - - - - 141

Prevention and Control Strategies - - - - 145
Bioterrorism - - - - - - - 165

OCCUPATIONAL HEALTH PROGRAMS

Screening and Immunization - - - - - 173
Staff Training and Counseling - - - - - 175
Occupational Health Administration - - - - 177

LEADERSHIP, MANAGEMENT AND COMMUNICATION

Leadership and Management - - - - 179
Communication - - - - - - 187
Planning - - - - - - - - 201

EDUCATION

Health Education - - - - - - - 207
Education Research - - - - - - 225

PRACTICE EXAMINATION

Multiple-Choice Quiz - - - - - - 235
Answer Key - - - - - - - - 283

ABOUT TRIVIUM TEST PREP

Trivium Test Prep uses industry professionals with decades worth of knowledge in the fields they have mastered, proven with degrees and honors in law, medicine, business, education, military, and more to produce high-quality test prep books such as this for students.

Our study guides are specifically designed to increase ANY student's score, regardless of his or her current scoring ability. At only 25% - 35% of the page count of most study guides, you will increase your score, while significantly decreasing your study time.

HOW TO USE THIS GUIDE

This guide is not meant to reteach you material you have already learned or waste your time on superfluous information. We hope you use this guide to focus on the key concepts you need to master for the test and develop critical test-taking skills. To support this effort, the guide provides:

- Practice questions with worked-through solutions
- Key test-taking tactics that reveal the tricks and secrets of the test
- Simulated one-on-one tutor experience
- Organized concepts with detailed explanations
- Tips, tricks, and test secrets revealed

Because we have eliminated "filler" or "fluff", you will be able to work through the guide at a significantly faster pace than other prep books. By allowing you to focus ONLY on those concepts that will increase your score, study time is more effective and you are less likely to lose focus or get mentally fatigued.

INTRODUCTION

THE CERTIFICATION BOARD OF INFECTION CONTROL AND EPIDEMIOLOGY (CBIC®) EXAM

The Certification Board of Infection Control and Epidemiology is an interdisciplinary board that administers the certification process for professionals in infection control and applied epidemiology.

CBIC'S VISION STATEMENT

CBIC provides professional certification for persons who work in infection prevention and control. CBIC Certification helps infection prevention and control professionals ensure the quality of care that the public expects, demands, and deserves.

CBIC is accredited by the National Commission on Certifying Agencies, a committee of the National Competency Assessment Organization.

THE CBIC'S MISSION STATEMENT

From the CBIC Web Site[1]: "The mission of CBIC is to protect the public through the development, administration, and promotion of an accredited certification in infection prevention and control."

STANDARDS OF PRACTICE FOR INFECTION CONTROL PROFESSIONALS

Although the CBIC puts forth no standards of practice, other regulatory and professional bodies such as the Centers for Disease Control and Prevention (CDC) and the Association for Professionals in

---

[1] cbic.org

Infection Control and Epidemiology (APIC) have developed standards of practice.

CDC STANDARDS OF PRACTICE

On their website[2], the CDC has published standards of practice regarding:

- Prevention of intravascular catheter-related infections
- Prevention and control of norovirus gastroenteritis outbreaks
- Prevention of catheter-associated urinary tract infections
- Control of infections with carbapenem-resistant or carbapenemase-producing Enterobacteriaceae in acute care facilities
- Public reporting of healthcare-associated infections
- Disinfection and sterilization in healthcare facilities
- Isolation precautions in hospitals
- A guide for management of multidrug resistant organisms in healthcare settings (2006)
- Preventing the transmission of Mycobacterium tuberculosis in healthcare facilities
- Preventing healthcare-associated pneumonia
- Infection control in dental healthcare settings
- Environmental infection control in healthcare facilities
- Hand hygiene in healthcare settings
- Prevention of surgical site infection

---

[2] cdc.gov

- Recommendations for preventing the spread of vancomycin resistance

APIC STANDARDS OF PRACTICE

On their website[3], the APIC has published standards of practice. According to these standards, the infection control professional:

1. Incorporates into practice effective activities that are specific to the practice setting, the population served, and the continuum of care

    - Integrates surveillance findings into formal plans for improvement of practice and patient outcomes in various health care settings; reviews; analyzes; and implements regulations, standards, and/or guidelines of applicable governmental agencies and professional organizations

    - Integrates relevant local, national, and global public health issues into practice

    - Analyzes and applies pertinent information from current scientific literature and publications

    - Develops and implements policies and procedures based on currently accepted infection prevention and control best practices

    - Ensures that findings, recommendations, and policies of the program are disseminated to appropriate groups or individuals

    - Provides knowledge on the function, role, and value of the program to customers.

2. Uses a systematic surveillance approach to monitor the effectiveness of prevention and control strategies that are consistent with the organization's goals and objectives.

---

[3] apic.org

- Develops a surveillance plan based on the population(s) served, services provided, and previous surveillance data

- Selects indicators and designs surveillance based on the projected use of the data

- Integrates pertinent regulatory requirements

- Uses standardized definitions for the identification and classification of events, indicators, or outcomes

- Utilizes information technology and systems applications

- Reports epidemiologically significant findings to appropriate customers

- Ensures requirements for communicable disease reporting are met

- Periodically evaluates the effectiveness of the surveillance plan and modifies as necessary

3. Applies epidemiologic principles and statistical methods, including risk stratification and benchmarking, to identify target populations, determine risk factors, design prevention and control strategies, analyze trends, and evaluate processes.

    - Uses epidemiologic principles to conduct surveillance and investigations

    - Employs statistical techniques to describe the data, calculate risk-adjusted rates, and benchmark

    - Incorporates information technology and systems applications in the analysis and dissemination of data

    - Critically evaluates significance of findings and makes recommendations for improvement based on those findings

4. Serves as an educator and educational resource for health care providers, ancillary staff, patients, families, and the general public.

    - Assesses the needs of customers and develops educational objectives and strategies to meet those needs
    - Utilizes learning principles appropriate to the target audience
    - Utilizes appropriate information technology in educational design and delivery
    - Collaborates in the development and delivery of educational programs and/or tools that relate to infection prevention, control, and epidemiology
    - Evaluates the effectiveness of educational programs and learner outcomes

5. Provides expert knowledge and guidance in infection prevention, control, and epidemiology.

    - Stays current with developments in infection prevention, control, and epidemiology
    - Integrates into practice, policies, and procedures, pertinent regulatory requirements; accreditation standards; and guidelines
    - Supports patients/families, administration, committees, health care providers and ancillary staff

IDENTIFYING INFECTIOUS DISEASES

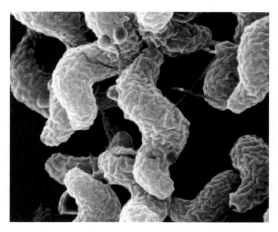

In this section, you will find details on the disease process and the chain of infection, as well as information about occurrences, reservoirs, incubation periods, periods of communicability, modes of transmission, signs and symptoms and susceptibility. This will provide a framework for your continuing studies of infection control and epidemiology.

TERMINOLOGY

According to the CDC, these are the basic terms and terminology relating to infections and infection control:

- **Administrative controls** are the use of administrative measures like enforcement measures, policies and procedures that are designed to reduce the risks of pathogenic transmissions in the health care setting. An example of an administrative control is a policy and procedure related to the disposal of sharps and other bio-hazardous waste.

- **Aerosols** are small particles less than 10 ! m that can remain airborne and viable for extended periods of time in the environment. Aerosols are most commonly produced and generated by things like water and air syringes.

- **Airborne transmission** is the mode and means of transmission for a pathogen that is airborne and then possibly inhaled by the host as droplet nuclei.

- **Alcohol-based hand rub** is an alcohol-containing preparation designed for reducing the number of viable microorganisms on the hands. These rubs are not a substitute for good hand washing and they are only to be used when hand washing facilities and materials are not available.

- **Allergen** is an antigen which can cause hypersensitivity and an allergic reaction in the host. Hosts can have sensitivity to medications, foods and other environmental sources like toxins.

- **Allergic contact dermatitis** is swelling or irritation of the skin that results from contact with a chemical. It is often localized to the area of the body that touched the contaminated item, which occurs slowly over twelve to forty eight hours after direct contact. Some examples of chemicals that can lead to allergic contact dermatitis include latex or another component in gloves, as well as plants like poison ivy and poison oak.

- **Anaphylaxis** is a severe and life threatening allergic response that occurs during exposure to an allergen like penicillin, latex in gloves and some pollens. The first exposure or dose is referred to as the sensitizing exposure or dose; the second exposure or dose is the one that leads to anaphylaxis, or anaphylactic shock. The signs and symptoms of anaphylaxis are hives, itching, respiratory problems, anaphylactic shock, coma and in some cases, death.

- **Antibodies** are proteins in the blood produced as the result of exposure to an antigen or pathogen. Antibodies bind to antigens and destroy them. Many vaccines produce antibodies to specific infections, giving a person protective immunity against a pathogen or infectious agent.

- **Antigens** are a protein or carbohydrate substance that enters the body and activates the immune process by stimulating the production of protective antibodies.

- **Antiseptic** is a germicidal solution that can be used to inhibit the growth of microorganisms, including pathogens, or to destroy it. Some examples of antiseptics include hexachlorophene, iodine, alcohol and antiseptic hand washes.

- **Asepsis** is a method used to prevent the spread of infection. The two types of asepsis are medical asepsis, or clean procedure, and surgical/sterile asepsis.

- **Bacterial count** is an estimation of the number of organisms in a unit of measurement. Bacterial counts are usually determined in terms of colony-forming-units per square centimeter/per milliliter.

- **Bio-burden** is the number of viable microorganisms on a surface or an object prior to decontamination and/or sterilization. Bio-burden is also referred to as microbiological load, microbial load and bio-load.

- **Biological indicators** are devices used to monitor the effectiveness of sterilization processes, in terms of whether these processes effectively destroy microorganisms and spores.

- **Blood-borne pathogens** are disease-producing pathogens that are spread and transmitted to others via contact with blood and other bodily fluids. Some examples of blood-borne pathogens are HIV and hepatitis.

- **Blood-borne Pathogens Standard** is a legal and binding regulation mandates that all employers protect their staff from occupational exposures to infectious agents and pathogens.

- **Chemical indicators** are a device used to monitor the effectiveness of sterilization processes in terms of whether these processes meet the rigors of effectiveness. Chemical indicators change their color or their form when they are exposed to sterilization temperatures and pressures. These indicators, like biological indicators, can alert personnel that there has been an error or malfunction in terms of packaging, cleaning, decontamination, sterilizer loading and a breakdown of the equipment itself.

- **Chemical sterilants** are chemicals able to destroy all microorganisms and bacterial spores.

- **Cleaning** is the physical, manual removal of visible material from a device or surface using scrubbing, water and a detergent or surfactant. Cleaning can also be done using an appropriate solution and an ultrasonic cleaner.

- **Colony Forming Unit (CFU):** is the minimum number of separable cells on or in an agar that creates a colony. A colony can be comprised of single cells, clusters of cells, chains and pairs of cells. These units of measurement are expressed as colony-forming-units per milliliter, or CFU/ml.

- **Contaminated** means having been in contact with a microorganism. Sterile items are contaminated when sterile technique is not scrupulously followed. Clean or medically aseptic items are contaminated when they have not been managed and handled in a manner that preserves medical asepsis.

- **Critical medical devices** are medical instruments or devices used to enter the body or the bloodstream, both of which are sterile areas of the body. Critical medical devices are typically used for invasive procedures, all of which are risky in terms of the introduction of infection. Examples of critical medical devices are intravenous catheters, indwelling urinary catheters, scalpels and endoscopes.

- **Decontamination** is, according to OSHA[4], defined as "the use of physical or chemical means to remove, inactivate, or destroy blood-borne pathogens on a surface or item to the point where they are no longer capable of transmitting infectious particles and the surface or item is rendered safe for handling, use, or disposal."

- **Direct contact transmission** is a mode of transmission in which there is a physical transfer of microorganisms between a colonized or infected person and a host.

- **Disinfectants** are chemical agents used on nonliving surfaces and items that will destroy most pathogens, but not endospores.

---

[4] osha.gov/pls/oshaweb/owadisp.show_document?p_id=10051&p_table=STANDARDS

- **Disinfection:** is the destruction of microorganisms, including pathogens, using a chemical or physical means of disinfection. Although disinfection destroys most pathogens, disinfection does not destroy spores.

- **Droplet nuclei** are minute particles less than 5μm diameter that can be transported and carried in the air for relatively long periods of time.

- **Droplets** are small particles of moisture from sprays and splatters. Some examples of droplets include particles propelled when a person coughs or sneezed and particles that are spread with a splatter of blood. Droplets do not last as long as droplet nuclei in the air, therefore, they are less hazardous in terms of transmission most typically affect those in close proximity to the source spray or splatter.

- **Endotoxins** are the lipopolysaccharides of gram-negative bacteria that can lead to pyrogenic reactions.

- **Engineering Controls**, like administrative and work practice controls, aim to prevent the transmission of healthcare pathogens and infections. Some examples of engineering controls include needleless systems and impervious labeled sharps disposal containers.

- **Event-related packaging** is the storage method that deems packages and contents sterile until some event, like moisture, saturates the item and renders it contaminated.

- **Exposure time** is the duration that an item is subjected to the disinfection or sterilization process.

- **Germicide** is an agent that destroys microorganisms including pathogens. These agents include antiseptics, which are used on human skin, and disinfectants that are used on inanimate objects in the environment.

- **Healthcare Associated Infection (HAI)** is any infection that is the result of a medical or surgical intervention in the healthcare setting.

- **Hepatitis B Immune Globulin (HBIG)** provides artificial, passive, temporary immunity of about three to six months against the hepatitis B virus.

- **Hepatitis B Surface Antigen (HBsAg)** is a serologic marker that, when elevated, indicates chronic or acute hepatitis B.

- **Hepatitis B e Antigen (HBeAg)** is also found in serum during acute and chronic hepatitis infection and it is indicative of viral replication and increasing infection.

- **Hepatitis B Surface Antibody (anti-HBs)** is the protective antibody against the hepatitis B virus (HBsAg). When this is present in the blood, it is indicative of a past infection, immunity to hepatitis B or an anticipated immune response after immunization with the hepatitis B vaccine.

- **High-level disinfection** is the process of inactivating bacteria, mycobacteria, fungi, and viruses, but not large numbers of bacterial spores

- **Hypersensitivity** is an allergic immune response to an antigen.

- **Iatrogenic** infections and other complications result accidentally from a medical intervention or diagnostic procedure.

- **Immunity** is protection against a disease. Immunity can be active, passive, natural and artificial. Active immunity occurs when antibodies are created in response to an antigen; passive immunity occurs when the fetus gets immunity from the mother in utero or from the injection of an immune globulin. Natural immunity occurs when the person develops antibodies to an infection because they have been infected with it; and artificial immunity is acquired when the person has received an immunization against the infection.

- **Immunization** is the process by which a person becomes immune with an injection.

- **Indirect contact transmission** is the mode of transmission in which the host has contact with a contaminated inanimate object.

- **Intermediate level disinfection** is a disinfection process that, in contrast to high level disinfection, deactivates vegetative bacteria, most fungi, mycobacteria, and most viruses, but not bacterial spores.

- **Low-level disinfection** is a disinfection process that deactivates most vegetative bacteria, some fungi, and some viruses, but not resistant microorganisms (such as spores and mycobacteria).

- **Mechanical indicators** are sterilization devices like a gauge or meter that indicate, or display, the time, temperature and/or pressure during the sterilization process.

- **Medical regulated waste** is bio-hazardous waste that can cause infection without proper handling and disposal. Some examples of medical regulated waste include blood-soaked materials and sharp objects that have been used for surgery or another invasive procedure.

- **Noncritical medical devices** are medical items that pose the least amount of risk in terms of infection transmission when contrasted with critical medical devices. Some examples of noncritical medical devices include blood pressure cuffs and environmental surfaces such as floors and countertops.

- **Occupational exposure** is the exposure of a healthcare worker to an infectious organism that occurs during the course of work.

- **Opportunistic infections** are caused by a microorganism that does not ordinarily cause disease but is capable of doing so, under certain host conditions. Some of these conditions include HIV infection and other immunosuppressive diseases and disorders.

- **Particulate respirator:** a respirator that is used to protect healthcare workers from airborne pathogens such as tuberculosis. NIOSH approved respirators are custom fitted, fit-tested and maintained by the employer.

- **Personal protective equipment (PPE)** is specialized equipment and attire used by healthcare employees to protect against infections. Examples of personal protective equipment include gowns, gloves, goggles and respirators.

- **Post-exposure prophylaxis** is the prevention of infection after an individual has been exposed to an infectious agent. The administration of medications following an occupational exposure varies

- **Prevalence** is the number of new and existing disease cases among members of a population during a given period of time.

- **Prions** are protein particles without nucleic acid that can lead to a number of neurological diseases like Creutzfeldt-Jakob disease and Scrapie.

- **Resident flora** are natural microorganisms that reside in or on the human body without adverse effect. In fact, some natural flora are highly beneficial to life.

- **Semi-critical medical devices** are medical devices or instruments that come into contact with mucous membranes, but do not enter internal areas of the body. The other types of medical devices, as discussed above, are critical medical devices and noncritical medical devices according to the Spaulding classification of medical devices.

- **Sero-conversion** is the production of antibodies by a person who had no prior detectable antibodies.

- **Spaulding classification** is a category of medical devices and the degree of sterilization or disinfection that is needed. The three categories are critical medical devices, semi-critical medical devices and noncritical medical devices, as discussed above, that need three levels of high, intermediate, and low disinfection or sterilization, respectively.

- **Sterilants** are chemical germicides that destroy all forms of microbiological life, including high numbers of resistant bacterial spores.

- **Sterile/sterility** means free from all living microorganisms. In practice, usually described as a probability function, (e.g., the probability of a surviving microorganism being 1 in 1,000,000).

- **Sterilization** is the destruction of all microorganisms and large numbers of bacterial spores with the use of a chemical or physical sterilizer.

- **Surfactants** are agents that clean surfaces by reducing surface tension, emulsifying and loosening debris.

- **Transient flora** are microorganisms that are in or on the body only with certain conditions and limited periods of time.

- **Transmission-based precautions** are special measures and practices to prevent the spread of infection based on the manner in which microorganisms are transmitted. These special measures are in addition to standard precautions.

- **Work practice controls** are infection control preventive work practices that reduce the possibility of an occupational exposure to a pathogen. Some examples of work practice controls include the prohibition of recapping needles and the correct use of intravenous catheters. These controls, when incorporated into the everyday work routine, reduce the likelihood of exposure by altering the manner in which a task is performed (e.g., prohibiting recapping of needles by a two-handed technique).

HOW INFECTIONS WORK

COLONIZATION

Colonization is the presence of microorganisms on bodily surfaces and cavities like the mouth, intestines, skin and airway passage that are not causing disease or symptoms. Specifically, the patient has a high, detectable concentration of microorganisms at a site without adverse health effects. Colonies may, however, cause infections and symptoms when they gain entry into more sterile internal structures like the circulatory system's bloodstream, the lungs, the kidneys and the bladder.

When colonies invade the lungs or other sections of the respiratory tract, they can cause respiratory infections like streptococcus as well as respiratory signs and symptoms. When the colonization invades the urinary tract, signs, symptoms and infectious disease affect this bodily system. The general signs and symptoms of infection are fever, chills and malaise.

A carrier of an infectious disease is defined as a person that is asymptomatic but able to transmit the infectious disease to others. Periods of colonization vary according to the person's immune responses to the particular organization, the use of any antimicrobials and the competition of other microorganisms at the site. The duration of colonization can range from a few days to several years.

INFECTION

Infection is defined as the physical invasion of a pathogenic organism that leads to an infection and an immune response by the affected individual.

CONTAMINATION

Contamination can refer to a number of different settings and processes. For example, sterile equipment is contaminated when sterile procedure is breached. With this situation, the sterility of the item is no longer ensured and, although it is not "dirty" or grossly contaminated, the item itself is still considered contaminated. The same is true for "clean" items that are processed and managed with medical asepsis. For example, clean latex gloves become contaminated once they touch a bodily surface or another "non-clean" surface.

Contamination also refers to reservoirs such as water and foods that are contaminated with infectious material.

THE CHAIN OF INFECTION

The chain of infection reflects the manner with which infections are transmitted and carried. The elements in the chain of infection include the agent, the reservoir, the environment, the mode of transmission, the portal of entry, the portal of exist and the susceptible host.

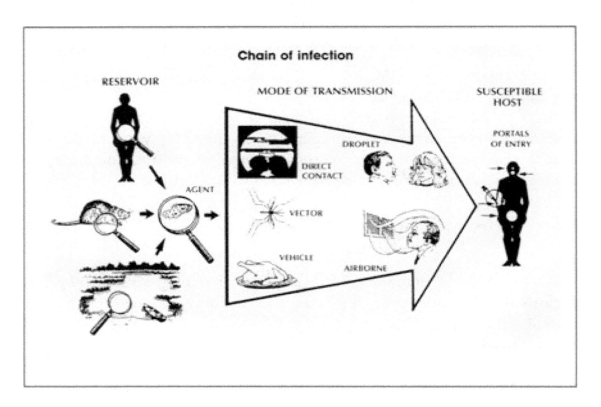

CAUSATIVE AGENTS

There are a wide variety of microorganisms that can cause infections and diseases among humans and there are also a wide variety of microorganisms that do not lead to infections and diseases. There are also some microorganisms that are highly beneficial to humans in terms of health. It is the pathogenic, or disease-causing, agents that infection control aims to eliminate.

The ability of a pathogenic microorganism to cause disease depends on a number of factors, including pathogenicity, virulence and the infective dose.

PATHOGENICITY

Pathogenicity is defined as the ability of the agent to cause disease. It is quantified as the ratio of people who develop disease out of the total number exposed to it.

VIRULENCE

How severe and intense the microbe is. Some are highly virulent and others have a low level of virulence.

INFECTIVE DOSE

The infective dose refers to the amount of the agent necessary to lead to infection. Some agents need a higher dosage than others in order to infect the person.

BACTERIA

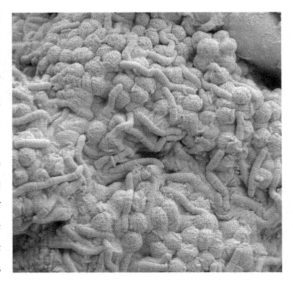

Bacteria can be categorized and classified in several ways including their morphology and their reactions to some laboratory tests. Bacteria are single-cell beings that appear as spirals, rods, spheres and other shapes. Some are pathogenic, lead to disease and release tissue damaging toxins; others are highly beneficial to the body. Some examples of bacteria include streptococcus, staphylococcus and E. coli.

Bacterial shapes and morphologies include spherical or round shapes (cocci), spiral shaped (spirochetes), rod-shaped (bacilli), and even cubes and tetrahedral shapes. They also form and cluster into different formations.

Some bacteria are classified as gram-positive because they react to a gram stain; these microbes have thick walls containing teichoic acid and peptidoglycan. Others are classified as gram-negative because they do not react to a gram stain. These microbes, more common than gram-positive bacteria, have thinner walls comprised of peptidoglycan and a lipid membrane, which includes endotoxins like lipoproteins and lipopolysaccharides.

Bacteria are also differentiated by their ability to resist color changes when subjected to other staining procedures in the laboratory. Acid-fast bacteria resist decolorization when stained with a Ziehl-Neelsen or Kinyoun stain, for example.

BACTERIAL GROWTH

The four phases of bacterial growth are the lag phase, the log phase, the stationary phase and the death phase, in this sequential order.

The lag phase of bacterial growth is characterized with the bacteria's acclamation to the new environment and a period of slow growth. The rate of biosynthesis is high because the bacteria need these proteins for future, rapid growth.

- *The log phase*, often referred to as the exponential phase, consists of a period of rapid and continuous growth until one or more of the nutrients needed to grow is exhausted.
- *The stationary stage*, which results from depleted nutrients, is marked with a halt in growth and metabolic activity.
- *The death stage* is the end of the bacteria's life. There are no nutrients left.

VIRUSES

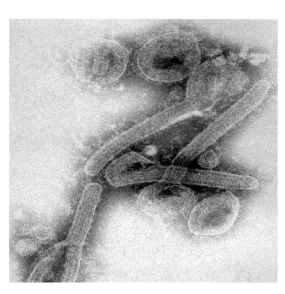

Viruses, which are much smaller than bacteria, have three parts including RNA, DNA and long molecules which comprise its genetic composition, the protein coat and an outer coating that contains lipids.

Viruses can have a wide host range and be capable of infecting many species, or a narrow host range that limits it to only some species.

Viruses, like bacteria, can be categorized and classified in several ways. For example, they can be categorized according to the host cell that they can infect. Viruses can be plant viruses, fungal viruses and animal viruses. They can also be classified according to their shape. Viruses come in several shapes including icosahedral and helical shapes, as well as more intricate and complex forms. They can also be categorized according to their nucleic acid composition and their method of replication. These classifications are:

- *DNA viruses*, which include both single and double-stranded DNA viruses.

- *RNA viruses,* which include single and double-stranded RNA viruses, negative sense and positive sense viruses.

- *Reverse transcribing viruses* including double-stranded reverse transcribing DNA viruses, single-stranded reverse transcribing RNA viruses and retroviruses.

The six stages of virus growth are attachment, penetration, un-coating, replication, self-assembly and release, in that sequential order.

- *The attachment stage* occurs when the virus attaches to a receptor on the host's cellular surface. Some are very specific and limited in terms of their abilities to attach; as such, they have a low or limited host range.

- *The penetration stages* occur when the virus enters the host's cell. This process is also referred to as viral entry.

- *The un-coating phase* involves the removal of the viral capsid, or coating, thus allowing the virus's nucleic material into the host cell.

- *The replication stage* is characterized with the replication and multiplication of the genome.

- *The self-assembly phase* follows the replication stage. During this phase, the maturation and modifications of the viral proteins occur.

- *The release of the virus* from the host cells, with lysis, occurs during this stage. Now, the cell is killed with this lysis.

FUNGI

There are an enormous number of fungi in our natural environment, including those in the soil, in plant life and on human beings. Fortunately, the vast majority of fungi are harmless; however, there are some that can lead to serious infections among humans, particularly when they are immunocompromised.

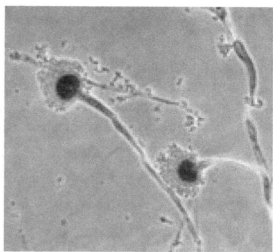

Fungi have mutualistic, antagonist, and commensal symbiotic relationships with other organisms, including humans.

- *Mutualistic* symbiotic relationships benefit both the virus and the organism it is attached to

- *Antagonistic* symbiotic relationships harm the fungi's host

- *Commensal* symbiotic relationships neither harm nor benefit the fungus or the host.

Although fungi in the world of botany can be categorized and classified in many ways, fungi that affect human beings are typically classified as superficial, cutaneous, subcutaneous and systemic.

- *Superficial fungal infections* affect the skin's epidermis and the hair. These infections can often occur among healthy people. An example of a superficial fungal infection is tinea capitis, which is often referred to as ringworm of the scalp, because it takes on the appearance of a worm despite the fact that it is caused by a fungus.

- *Cutaneous fungal infections* include invasive hair and nail infections that go beyond the epidermis. An example of a cutaneous fungal disease is athlete's foot, or tinea pedis.

- *Subcutaneous fungal infections* can infect all layers of the skin to the muscles and the fascia. These fungal infections, often serious, typically result from a deep puncture wound.

- *Systemic fungi infections* are typically highly virulent and hey can spread to virtually all organs of the body. Those with immunosuppression as the result of HIV, chemotherapy and metastatic cancer are at greatest risk. Some examples of systemic fungal infections include aspergillosis, candidiasis and cryptococcosis.

PRIONS

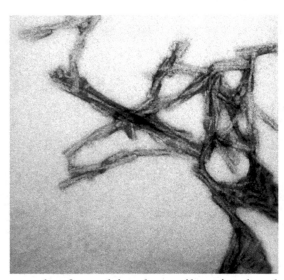

A prion is not a living organism; it is defined as an abnormal folding of normal cellular, or prion, proteins. Some of the infectious diseases associated with prions include encephalopathy, including Creutzfeldt-Jakob ("mad cow" disease) and other rare diseases such as kuru, or fatal familial insomnia. It is currently believed that humans become infected when they ingest teprion, which can be found in the soil or in dead animals.

Prions and prion diseases primarily affect the brain and neural tissue; these infections are associated with a high morbidity and mortality rate without a possible cure. Prions can be destroyed only with sterilization.

PARASITES

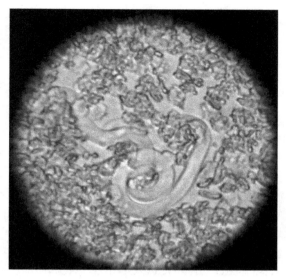

A parasite is an organism that lives on or in a host and gets its food from or at the expense of its host. Parasites can cause disease in humans. Some parasitic diseases are easily treated and some are not. The burden of these diseases often rests on communities in the tropics and subtropics, but parasitic infections can also affect people in developed countries. Some examples of parasitic infections include giardia, tapeworms, pin worms, lice infestations, maggot infestation and scabies.

GIARDIA

Giardia infection, known as giardiasis, is caused by a microscopic parasite that is most commonly found in areas with poor sanitation and unsafe water. This infection is waterborne, and can be found anywhere from back country streams or lakes to swimming pools and spas. It is also transmitted through food and person-to-person contact.

Signs and Symptoms

In some cases, people with the infection are just carriers, but they can still infect others that come in contact with their stool. The symptoms include watery, foul smelling diarrhea, fatigue, malaise, abdominal cramps and bloating, nausea, weight loss, and belching gas with a bad taste. Symptoms usually last for two to four weeks.

Treatment

Mild cases usually go away automatically; severe cases are treated with antibiotic medications, such as metronidazole, tinidazole and nitazoxanide.

TAPEWORMS

Tapeworm infestation occurs when food or water is contaminated with tapeworm eggs or larvae. Invasive infection occurs when the tapeworm eggs migrate outside of the intestines and form larval cysts in bodily tissue or organs.

An intestinal infection is one in which tapeworm larvae are ingested but develop into adult tapeworms in the intestines. The adult tapeworm, which can live for 20 years, consists of a head, neck and chain of segments, which are called proglottids. The head adheres to the intestine and the proglottids grow and produce eggs. Intestinal infections are usually mild, but an invasive larva infection can be quite serious.

Signs and Symptoms

Intestinal tapeworms usually cause no signs and symptoms, but if they do they include nausea, weakness, loss of appetite, abdominal pain, diarrhea, and weight loss and an inadequate absorption of nutrients from food.

Invasive infections, in which the larvae have migrated out of the intestines and have formed cysts in other tissues, can eventually lead to organ and tissue damage. Symptoms include fever, allergic reactions to the larvae, bacterial infections, cystic masses or lumps, and neurological symptoms such as seizures.

Treatment

Many types of ringworm will exit the body on their own, while others need treatment. Medications, such as praziquantel, albendazole, and nitazoxanide are toxic to ringworms. Reinfection may occur, so follow-up stool samples are taken, and education on hand washing is given.

For invasive infections, depending on the location and effects of the infection, antihelmintic drugs, such as albendazole. may be used to shrink the cyst. If the tapeworm is dying, anti-inflammatory therapy and corticosteroids, such as prednisone or dexamethasone, may be indicated. Seizures from the disease can be treated with anticonvulsant medications.

PINWORMS

Pinworms are the most common type of intestinal worm in the U.S. They are thin, white, and measure about 5 to 13 millimeters in length. This infestation is most common among school age children.

Signs and Symptoms

Some people have no symptoms, but those who do may experience itching of the anus or vaginal area, insomnia or restlessness, pain and nausea.

Treatment

Those with no symptoms may not need treatment, but those with them may be prescribed an antiparasite medication, such as mebendazole or albendazole. Often times the medication is given to all the members of the household to prevent both the spread of the infection and reinfection.

LICE

Lice are tiny, parasitic insects that feed on blood. Lice can be found on the head, the body, and the pubic area, which are referred to commonly as "crabs".

Signs and Symptoms

Signs and symptoms include intense itching and small, red bumps on the scalp, neck and shoulders. Adult lice are about the size of a sesame seed and the nits resemble dandruff.

Treatment

Treatment for head lice includes a special over-the-counter shampoo, malathion, benzyl alcohol lotion or lindane.

MAGGOT INFESTATION OR MYIASIS

Myiasis is classified according to the area affected. These classifications include dermal, sub dermal, cutaneous, nasopharyngeal, ocular, auricular, gastrointestinal and urogenital myiasis.

Signs and Symptoms

- *Aural Myiasis*: The patient may report buzzing in their ear. Ear discharge, if present, may be foul smelling. The larvae can enter the brain when the middle and inner ear are affected.

- *Cutaneous Myiasis*: Painful boils that can last for an extensive period of time.

- *Ophthalmomyiasis*: Eye irritation, pain and edema

- *Nasal Myiasis*: Nasal congestion and obstruction, fever, and facial edema

Treatment

The surgical removal of the larva is done with a local anesthetic such as lidocaine, and forceps. After removal, the site is dressed and antibiotics are often given to prevent a secondary infection. Another treatment, although not preferred, occludes and suffocates the larva.

Cutaneous myiasis is treated with a thick coat of petroleum jelly to rob the larva of their oxygen supply, which then moves them to the surface for relatively simple removal. All types of myiasis can be treated with oral ivermectin (200 mcg/kg) ivermectin or topical ivermectin (1% solution).

SCABIES

An itchy skin condition caused by *Sarcoptes scabiei*, a tiny burrowing mite, is known as scabies. This condition is contagious and can it can spread quickly.

Signs and Symptoms

The signs and symptoms include itchiness, often worse at night, thin, irregular burrow tracks made up of tiny blisters or bumps on the skin. In adults it is mostly found between fingers, in armpits, on the inner elbow, soles of the feet, around breasts, around male genital area, along the insides of wrists, and around the waist. In children, it is commonly seen on the scalp, face, neck, palms of the hands and soles of the feet.

Treatment

Treatment includes medications, such as permethrin 5%, lindane, and crotamiton. In some cases the oral medication ivermectin is used for those who do not respond to the prescription lotions and creams.

RESERVOIRS AND TRANSMISSION

The reservoir, a part of the cycle of infection, is defined as the environment or habitat within which the pathogen lives, grows and reproduces. Reservoirs can include humans, animals, water, soil and insects.

HUMAN RESERVOIRS

The vast majority of infections that affect human beings have humans as their reservoir. Humans who serve as reservoirs may or may not be adversely affected with infection despite the fact that they serve as the habitat for the pathogen. For example, asymptomatic carriers are not adversely affected with the infection but they can still transmit it to others; those in the incubation period who have not yet developed the infection can still serve as the reservoir for the infectious agent.

There are also human reservoirs that can still transmit the infection to others despite the fact that the carrier has recovered from the infection; these people are referred to as convalescent carriers. There are also chronic carriers, like Typhoid Mary, who are chronic reservoirs capable of infecting others. Many reservoir carriers are not even aware of the fact that they can infect others.

ANIMAL RESERVOIRS

Humans are also susceptible to infection from animal reservoirs, although not to the same extent as human reservoirs.

Some animal reservoirs include cows (brucellosis), rodents (plague), pigs (trichinosis), sheep (anthrax), rabbits (tularemia), dogs and bats (rabies), and birds (West Nile encephalitis). Other diseases that have originated in animals reservoirs include HIV/AIDS, Ebola and Severe Acute Respiratory Syndrome (SARS), which is a viral respiratory infection.

SOIL RESERVOIRS

Many fungal agents, such as those that cause histoplasmosis, live and multiply in soil.

WATER RESERVOIRS

Safe drinking water is a global public health concern. Contaminated water is often the reservoir for a number of parasites. Some of the infections associated with water reservoirs include amebiasis, Legionnaires disease, cryptosporidiosis, schistosomiasis and giardiasis.

THE MODES OF TRANSMISSION

A mode of transmission, or transportation, which is part of the cycle of infection, allows a pathogen to move from its reservoir to its susceptible host. There are several modes of transmission including direct, indirect, airborne, vehicle and vector modes of transmission.

DIRECT TRANSMISSION

Direct transmission can occur through direct contact with the pathogen and with the spread of an infectious droplet. Depending on the pathogen, direct contact can occur with skin, mucous membrane contact as well as from contract with infectious material such as soil or water.

Droplet spread consists of direct contact with a spray of infectious material, which can occur as the result of coughing and even speaking. Examples of pathogens that spread through direct contact include parasitic diseases such as tapeworm, childhood diseases like pertussis and others, such as mononucleosis.

INDIRECT TRANSMISSION

This mode of transmission involves the movement of an infectious agent from the reservoir to the host by inanimate objects.

AIRBORNE TRANSMISSION

This type of transmission occurs when the pathogen is carried in dust or droplets in the air that remain in place long enough to infect someone who is exposed. Measles is an example of a virus that transports by the airborne mode of transmission.

VEHICLE TRANSMISSION

Vehicle transmissions occur when a person comes into contact with an infectious product that is in water, blood, and even inanimate objects like a toy or a doorknob.

VECTOR TRANSMISSION

Vectors, unlike vehicles, are live beings (such as ticks and mosquitoes) that spread infections by relatively direct mechanical means, like an insect bite.

PROTECTIVE PRECAUTIONS

These include:

- *Standard precautions,* which apply to all blood and bodily fluids, and all patients regardless of the person's diagnosis
- *Contact precautions,* which prevent any direct and indirect contact transmissions, like those contained in diarrhea, wounds, and herpes simplex.

- *Airborne precautions* are indicated for the prevention of airborne transmission microbes like TB. These include a HEPA mask and a negative pressure room.

- *Droplet precautions* are used to prevent the transmission of pathogens through a cough or sneeze. Masks are indicated for these precautions.

PORTALS OF ENTRY AND EXIT

PORTAL OF ENTRY

The portal of entry is the "open door" through which the pathogen enters the susceptible host and comes in contact with an environment that is favorable to their reproduction and growth. The portal of entry is most often identical to the portal of exit. For example, hepatitis B and C use the blood and other bodily fluids as both their portal of entry and their port of exit.

The most common portals of entry include the respiratory tract, through a droplet of airborne mode of transmission, the gastrointestinal tract, with transmission via the fecal-oral route, through the skin and mucous membranes, with direct contact, and the blood and other bodily fluids using these portals of entry as their same portal of exit.

PORTAL OF EXIT

In contrast to the portal of entry, this is the "exit door" by which the pathogen leaves the body. The portal of exit is often identical to the portal of entry.

THE SUSCEPTIBLE HOST

The last part of the chain of infection is the susceptible host. Simply defined, a susceptible host is a person unable to resist infection when exposed to it. Many factors affect susceptibility; some are related to the pathogen, and others are specific to the host. For example, it takes a higher level of susceptibility to resist a pathogen that is highly virulent with a high level of pathogenicity. Factors that affect the individual's susceptibility to infections include:

- *Age*: Infants and older adults are at greatest risk.

- *Heredity*: Many genetic factors increase the risk for infection, though others protect against them.

- *Level of stress*: Stress increases cortisol levels and elevated cortisol levels decrease the person's resistance to infections and their responsiveness in terms of anti-inflammatory responses.

- *Nutritional status*: People are more susceptible to infection when they have a poor nutritional status, particularly when they have a protein deficiency.

- *Current medications and treatments*: Treatments such as radiation therapy for cancer add to the person's susceptibility to infections. Medications like corticosteroids and antineoplastic cancer drugs decrease the person's immune responses, thus placing them at greater risk for infection than others without these medications and treatments.

- *The presence of diseases and other preexisting conditions*: All diseases and disorders that decrease the person's defenses against infection increase the person's susceptibility to infections. For example, diseases and disorders such as diabetes mellitus, HIV and peripheral vascular disease increase the person's susceptibility to infections.

RISK

Risk is defined as the probability that an infection will occur more often in one person or group than another. Some of the factors that contribute to a person's risk include susceptibility and exposure potential.

For example, a host's susceptibility to HIV increases when the host engages in risky sexual behavior. Exposure potential is a measure of how likely a person will come into contact with a pathogen. Healthcare workers have a greater exposure potential to blood-borne pathogens because of the nature of their job and their occupational exposures to sharps and bodily fluids.

BODILY DEFENSES AGAINST INFECTION

Some of the natural bodily defenses that protect humans from infection include nonspecific and specific defenses.

Some of the nonspecific defenses against infection include anatomical and physiological barriers to infection and the inflammation process itself.

Some of the specific responses to infection include the immune systems' antibody mediated defenses and the cell mediated defenses, or cellular immunity. Antibody mediated defenses include immunities, such as active immunity and passive immunity.

Active immunity is characterized by the production of antibodies in response to an antigen; passive immunity occurs when the host receives antibodies to the antigen in an artificial manner, such as immunization, or in a natural manner, as occurs when immunity is passed from mother to child in utero or during breastfeeding.

LEVELS OF PREVENTION

There are three prevention levels: Primary, secondary and tertiary.

PRIMARY

Primary prevention activities aim to prevent the occurrence of infection, disease and dysfunction before it actually occurs. Examples include:

- *Environmental Protection* - Some examples of primary prevention related to the environment include proper sanitation, clean water and a clean and uncontaminated food supply.

- *Health Promotion Activities* - Education and counseling are examples. For example, an infection control professional can educate and counsel individuals, groups and populations about the need for immunizations, hand washing and clean water in underserved, undeveloped geographic areas.

- *Immunizations* - Infection control professionals administer, or coordinate and plan, immunization programs for individuals like patients and staff members as well as groups and populations such as infants, young children and those at risk for infections such as influenza, pneumonia and shingles.

SECONDARY

Secondary prevention is designed to identify infections and other diseases at the earliest possible time so that they can be treated. Examples include:

- *Health Assessments for Individuals, Groups and Populations* - Infection control professionals perform complete and thorough assessments of individuals, groups of people and populations in order to determine things like risk factors, past medical history, strengths and weakness.

- *Immunizations* - Infection control professionals administer, or coordinate and plan, screening programs for individuals like patients and staff members as well as groups and populations such as infants, young children and those at risk for infections such as tuberculosis, for example. The purpose of this screening is to identify any infections at their earliest stages so they can be treated and/or prevented.

TERTIARY

Tertiary prevention aims to return the affected individual, group or population to the highest possible level of functioning after the correction of a health problem such as an infectious disease. Examples include:

- *Determining Compliance with Quarantine* - On rare occasions, individuals and groups are quarantined in order to protect the health and safety of others. Infection control professionals follow up with these individuals and groups to ensure that they remain quarantined until the threat has passed.

- *Determining Compliance with Medication Regimens* - Some medication regimens are long, prompting some patients to stop taking prescriptions for infections such as HIV and tuberculosis. Infection control follow-up is necessary to ensure compliance and to prevent complications.

THE IMPLICATIONS OF THE CHAIN OF INFECTION

The chain of infection reflects the manner in which infections are transmitted and carried. The elements in the chain of infection include the agent, the reservoir, the environment, the mode of transmission, the portal of entry, the portal of exit and the susceptible host.

All involved in infection control must be thoroughly knowledgeable about the cycle of infection in order to stop transmission by eliminating, or reducing, one or more of the links in the chain of infection. For example, the agent can be eliminated or reduced with proper hand washing and antibiotics for bacterial pathogens; the reservoir can be eliminated with sanitization of the drinking water supply; the mode of transmission can be rendered ineffective with the proper use of personal protective equipment such as a mask and isolation, or special precautions, when indicated; the portals of entry and exit can be controlled with a wide variety of infection control procedures including the use of bed nets to prevent the bite of an infectious mosquito that can spread West Nile virus;

and the susceptibility of the host can be increased with the maintenance of health and wellness and immunizations.

OCCURRENCE, INCUBATION AND COMMUNICABILITY

OCCURRENCES OF INFECTION

Occurrences are affected by a number of factors, including an increase in the number of infectious agents, an increase in the virulence of the agent, an enhanced mode of transmission, increases in the susceptibility of the host and the addition of new portals of entry and exit.

The occurrence of infection can be defined, described and measured in a number of different ways:

- **Rate** is the mathematical measurement of the frequency of an event that occurs in a specified period of time, and often in terms of a specific population. The rate of hospital-acquired infections, or nosocomial infections, may be expressed as the rate of two occurrences of hospital-acquired pneumonia during 100 days of hospitalization. Some rates commonly used in healthcare include birth rates, mortality rates and morbidity rates.

- **Incidence** is the mathematical number of *new* events, such as infections, in a specific population in a defined period. It is mathematically calculated as a percentage by dividing the number of new events per 1,000 or 10,000 people, or it can be simply expressed like 2: 1,000. The two most common measures of incidence are cumulative incidence rate and incidence density rate.

- **Prevalence** describes how widespread the occurrence of the infection is at a particular time. A prevalence rate is a proportion where the numerator (top number of the fraction) is the number of people with the infection, both new and existing, and the denominator (bottom number of the fraction) is the number of people who actually have the infection plus the number of people who are at risk for the infection.

Infection occurrences can also be described as epidemic, pandemic, endemic, syndemic and sporadic occurrences.

EPIDEMICS

An epidemic is defined as an infectious disease occurrence that is greater than expected. Epidemics occur for a number of reasons, but generally speaking, they are most common when there is a decrease in the host's immunity and/or an increase in the agent's, or infectious agents, numbers, virulence and/or pathogenicity.

Some epidemics can be seasonal. For example, the influenza and measles viruses predominantly occur during the winter months. Epidemics can be further classified as a common source outbreak or a propagated outbreak. Common source outbreaks, also referred to as a point source outbreak, occur when those affected with the infection had an exposure to the same, or common, agent. In a propagated outbreak, the infection is not spread with a pathogenic agent; instead, humans become infected with person-to-person contact. In a sense, the infected people are human reservoirs for the agent.

PANDEMICS

A pandemic is similar to an epidemic; however, pandemic infections are more widespread geographically than epidemics. Some examples of pandemics include HIV infection and other infectious diseases like smallpox and tuberculosis.

ENDEMIC

Endemic is the term used to describe either the constant and continuous presence or an unusual presence of an infectious agent in a particular geographic location. Hyperendemic is a persistent, continuous high level of infection occurrences in a particular geographic location.

SYNDEMIC

A syndemic is the combination of two diseases, or infections, that increases the negative effects of these infections as they and the hosts interact within the environment.

SPORADIC OCCURRENCES

Sporadic occurrences are irregular, rare outbreaks that are often unpredictable.

INCUBATION PERIODS

The incubation period is defined as the period of time that elapses between the initial exposure to the pathogen and the emergence of signs and symptoms. Some incubation periods can be quite brief and short, and others can be quite long. During this period, the pathogen establishes itself, goes to the target area(s) and begins to proliferate. In some cases, the latent period of the infection process may be shorter than the incubation period; in other cases, the latent period of the infection process may be longer than the incubation period. Although the latent period and the incubation period are similar, the latent period is the time between infection and infectiousness and the incubation period is the time between infection and the onset of the infection's signs and symptoms.

Some incubation periods are characterized by the ability of the host to infect others; other incubation periods can be noncontagious. A subclinical infection is a term that is sometimes used when a person can spread the infection, but the person has not yet had an onset of its signs and symptoms.

Incubation periods can be categorized as intrinsic incubation and extrinsic incubation periods. Intrinsic incubations are those which are marked by the time that the pathogen has had a chance to develop in the definitive host; extrinsic incubations reflect the amount of time that it takes for the pathogen to completely develop in the intermediate host.

Incubations and incubation periods are modified and impacted by many factors including individual variations, the route of entry, or exposure, the dose of the infectious agent, the host susceptibility to the pathogen and the rate of the infectious agent's replication rate. Generally speaking, incubation periods are shorter among infants and children and longer among the adult population.

PERIOD OF COMMUNICABILITY

The period of communicability is defined as the duration of time that a pathogen can indirectly or directly transmit an infection to another. This period of time varies according to the microorganism. Pathogens are characterized by brief and long periods of communicability.

THE STAGES OF INFECTION

These include:

- *The incubation stage*, which begins with the entry of the agent into the host and ends when the signs and symptoms of the infection begin.

- *The prodromal stage*, which begins with the onset of general symptoms and ends when infection specific symptoms begin. It is during the prodromal period that the pathogen is replicating and reproducing. Some of the general symptoms that appear during the prodromal phase include malaise, joint and muscular aches and pains, anorexia, and headache.

- *The illness stage* is the period of time when specific symptoms begin, and continues until the symptoms are no longer present.

- *The convalescence stage* is the period during which the symptoms disappear.

THE INFLAMMATORY PROCESS

The inflammatory process is a naturally occurring protective response of the body when it is affected by one of many possible causes of tissue damage. The goals of the inflammatory process are to defend against harm, to rid the body of damaged tissue and to promote the restoration of normal tissue.

The inflammatory process has five classical signs and symptoms:

- *Pain* results when chemicals are released from the damaged tissue and cells

- *Redness* occurs when the affected area vasodilates in response to injury

- *Swelling* occurs when bodily fluids go to the area of tissue damage

- *Heat and Warmth* occurs because blood flow to the area increases

- *Dysfunction* occurs when the area is painful and edematous

THE STAGES OF THE INFLAMMATORY PROCESS

The stages of the inflammatory process include:

- *Tissue injury* as the result of an infection or trauma

- *The release of chemicals* from the damaged cells, including histamine, prostaglandins and kinins, all of which facilitate vasodilation and an increased supply of blood

- *The migration of leukocytes*, including macrophages and neutrophils, to the site of damage, as part of the body's natural defense mechanisms

SIGNS AND SYMPTOMS OF INFECTION

The signs and symptoms of infection include both local and systemic signs.

The local signs of infection, like the signs and symptoms of the inflammatory process, are site pain, redness, heat, swelling and a degree of local dysfunction.

For example, respiratory infections are often characterized with a cough, dyspnea and adventitious breath sounds; urinary infections classically manifest with urinary frequency and urgency, dysuria and hematuria. Similarly, skin infections are typically marked with a rash, skin lesions and pruritus.

Some of the unusual and atypical signs of infection include confusion, incontinence and agitation. Additionally, the elderly may not present with the signs of infection as soon as younger patients, because their protective inflammatory response may be decreased due to their advanced age.

DIAGNOSTIC AND LABORATORY TESTS

BLOOD TESTS

Some of the commonly used blood laboratory tests for infections include the erythrocyte sedimentation rate (ESR), C-reactive protein (CRP) and plasma viscosity (PV). All of these tests are sensitive to increases in protein, which is a part of the inflammation process. The ESR, CRP and PV can be raised with primarily bacterial infections, abscesses and other disorders such as cancer, burns and a myocardial infarction. Some health problems like polycythemia, sickle cell anemia and heart failure are signaled by a less than normal ESR.

ERYTHROCYTE SEDIMENTATION RATE (ESR)

The erythrocyte sedimentation rate (ESR) measures the rate at which the red blood cells separate from the plasma and fall to the bottom of the test tube within a given period of time.

A high erythrocyte sedimentation rate indicates the presence of infection because the proteins of infection cover the red blood cells thus causing them to fall more rapidly.

The normal erythrocyte sedimentation rate (ESR) for females is 0-20 millimeters per hour and the normal rate for males is 0-15 millimeters per hour. The normal sedimentation rate among the elderly can be slightly higher.

C REACTIVE PROTEIN

C reactive protein, sometimes referred to as the acute phase of inflammation protein, can rise as high as 1000x above the normal rate when infection and inflammation occur. It can also rise with burns, surgery and cancer. The normal C reactive protein is < 1.0 mg/dL or less than 10 mg/L.

PLASMA VISCOSITY

Simply stated, blood viscosity is the thickness of the blood. Some of the factors that affect viscosity include plasma viscosity, hematocrit, the level of red blood cell aggregation and temperature. Higher temperatures lead to lower viscosity and lower temperatures lead to increase blood thickness and viscosity. The normal viscosity of the blood, at 37 °C, is 3×10^{-3} to 4×10^{-3}.

CULTURES AND SENSITIVITY TESTS

Cultures and sensitivity testing is frequently done for a wide variety of samples, including those relating to wound infections, gastrointestinal infections and urinary tract infections. When a culture and sensitivity is indicated, based on the patient's clinical condition, the sample is microscopically examined, after which it is cultured in an appropriate medium such as a nutrient broth or agar. Cultures are useful for the identification of the microorganism, to determine whether a wound, for example, is colonized or infected and also to get a numeric values for the colony. For example, a urine specimen may have 123 colony-forming units per mL (123 cfu/mL).

Sensitivity testing entails subjecting the culture to a number of different antibiotics in order to confirm whether or not the pathogen is treatable and sensitive to specific antibiotics, or whether it is resistant to the antibiotic, as is the case with methicillin-resistant Staphylococcus aureus (MRSA).

Specimens for microbiology, culture and sensitivity must be collected correctly and processed as soon as possible after collection, because some microorganisms may not survive prolonged lengths of time before the laboratory processes them.

URINE TESTS

More than 100 different tests can be performed on urine. A routine urinalysis measures the color, clarity, odor, specific gravity, pH, proteins, glucose, ketones, nitrites, leukocyte esterase and microscopic evaluation.

Bacteria can make normally clear urine cloudy. Infections can also make urine odorous. In the presence of a urinary tract infection, nitrites will be present and the leukocyte esterase will show white blood cells, or leukocytes in the urine.

Microscopic analysis is done after the urine is centrifuged to render sediment for analysis. Some of the things that can be found in urine with microscopic analysis include:

- Abnormal presence of red and/or white blood cells, which indicates inflammation and infection
- Casts, which also indicate infection
- Crystals in the presence of stones
- Bacteria, yeast, and/or parasites when an infection is present

SPINAL TAPS

Spinal taps, also referred to as a lumbar puncture, are performed to determine if the cerebrospinal fluid (CSF) is infected with meningitis. Normal CSF values are:

- A pressure of 70 - 180 mm H20
- A colorless and clear appearance
- 15 - 60 mg/100 mL of total protein
- 3 - 12% of the total protein is gamma globulin
- 50 - 80 mg/100 mL glucose
- 0 - 5 mononuclear white blood cells
- No red blood cells
- 110 - 125 mEq/L chloride

Increased CSF pressure occurs as the result of increased intracranial pressure. Protein can increase by an infection or any other inflammatory process, glucose can be decreased by infections like meningitis and tuberculosis, increased white blood cells can indicate an acute infection and red blood cells indicate bleeding.

DIAGNOSTIC IMAGING TESTS

A number of diagnostic imaging tests are used to diagnose infections:

- X-rays (used for illnesses like pneumonia)
- Computerized tomography (CT)
- Magnetic resonance imaging (MRI)
- Gallium scans can reveal infection when the radioactive gallium citrate accumulates in the area of infection and "hot spots" of white blood cells

BIOPSIES

Biopsies are not just used to diagnose cancer – they can also diagnose infections and inflammations caused by fungi, pneumonia and temporal arteritis.

LIMITATIONS AND ADVANTAGES OF TESTS TO DIAGNOSE INFECTIONS

All tests have limitations, advantages and disadvantages. Some tests are more effective than others for specific infections. Some are more costly and invasive than others. For example, endoscopic tests are more invasive and expensive than a blood or urine test. Additionally, some tests may have false negative and false positive findings. For these reasons, and others, diagnostic tests are a part of the diagnostic process and not the entire diagnostic process.

EPIDEMIOLOGY

Epidemiology is the study of how health-related states, such as illness and infection, are caused and distributed in specific populations. Epidemiology also encompasses the application of its research findings to controlling health problems.

THE EPIDEMIOLOGICAL PROCESS

The steps of the epidemiological process in correct sequential order are:

1. The definition of the problem or infectious situation

2. The description of the course or natural history of the event

3. The identification of points of control

4. The generation of possible strategies that can stop and/or reverse the course of the event

5. Deciding upon the strategies with the highest possibility of success

6. Designing ways with which these strategies can be implemented

7. Implementing these strategies

8. Evaluating the outcomes of these strategies in terms of their success and effectiveness

Epidemiology employs models such as the Epidemiological Triad (agent, host and environment), the Wheel of Causation, the Web of Causation, and the Determinants of Health Model.

THE EPIDEMIOLOGICAL TRIAD

The three components of Epidemiologic Triad, or triangle, are the agent, the host and the environment. The Epidemiologic Triad is dynamic and the three components are in a constant state of interaction with each other and with other factors like risk and the transmission of disease.

Some examples of agents, according to the Epidemiologic Triad, include chemical agents and infectious biological agents. Other factors that negatively impact on a patient's state of health include things like a genetic susceptibility to an infection or disease process, a state of immunocompromise and poor life style choices. Examples of environment factors included in the Epidemiologic Triad are things like a toxic environment, unclean water, unsafe food and hazardous working conditions.

THE WHEEL OF CAUSATION

The Wheel of Causation takes the focus away from the cause of the disease and places the emphasis on genetics as well as the biological, physical and social environments as the cause of disease.

THE WEB OF CAUSATION

The Web of Causation model moves further than the Epidemiological Triad and the Wheel of Causation, because the Web of Causation further describes the relationships and interrelationships among multiple factors that impact on health and disease, whereas the others do not continue to these more intricate and complex interrelationships.

THE DETERMINANTS OF HEALTH MODEL

This model recognizes that the intricate relationships among various and multiple factors impact on health and disease in a manner that is not simply two dimensional but instead multidimensional. The determinants of health are:

- *Human biological determinants* such as nutritional status and genetic composition

- *Psychological determinates* like stress, distress, anxiety and coping strategies

- *Social determinants* of health including cultural impacts and political structures

- *Economic determinants* like income status

- *Environmental determinants* like poor water quality

- *Health system determinants* like the accessibility of healthcare

- *Behavioral determinants* like lifestyle risk behaviors

DISEASE CAUSATION

Some theories of disease causation include factors such as bacteriological (HIV, rubella), psychological (stress), physical sources (heat, cold, trauma), environmental factors (water or air pollutants), genetic composition (sickle cell anemia), chemical agents (ammonia, medications) and other single causes, as well as multiple cause combinations.

The CDC identifies five factors, or criteria, that are necessary in order to establish a causal, or cause-effect, relationship, in terms of cause and the occurrence of infection. These five factors are:

- Plausibility
- Strength of association
- Consistency
- Temporality
- Biological gradient

The plausibility criteria require that the explanation makes sense biologically; the strength of the association requires that the relationship is a clear one. Consistency is present when the association is, and can be, observed repeatedly among different populations and at different times; and temporality requires that the cause must come before the effect. Lastly, there must be a dose response relationship, which is the biological gradient.

Some add two additional criteria to support causality. These criteria are scientific experimental evidence and the specificity of the association. The specificity of the association means that the disease, like an infectious disease, is caused by only one agent and that specific agent only causes this disease or disorder.

EPIDEMIOLOGICAL INVESTIGATION

Scientific inquiry and epidemiological investigation are essential components of epidemiology. There are several types of investigations, including descriptive, analytic, experimental and more.

Descriptive Investigations

Descriptive research explores and describes the distribution of health events, like infections and diseases, as related to personal characteristics, place or time (secular trends, point epidemic, event related clusters, and cyclical patterns) and a number of other variables.

Analytic Investigations

Analytical research explores the "why and how" of factors that affect health events or outcomes. For example, analytical research may seek to determine how epidemiological factors affect increases and decreases in the occurrence rate of events such as infectious illness.

Analytical investigations are performed by a number of research designs, all of which have advantages and disadvantages. These include:

- *Prospective cohort*, which employs concurrent data and longitudinal data

- *Retrospective cohort*, which employs the use of retrospective rather than concurrent data

- *A cross sectional or correlation study*

- *Ecologic studies*

- *Case control investigations* including case comparisons

Experimental Investigations

Experimental investigations are similar to analytical investigations and descriptive studies in that they observe exposures and the outcomes or events, but these investigations add the components of randomization and the introduction of some intervention that may alter the presence or level of the healthcare outcome/event.

MEASUREMENTS AND TOOLS

The best data measurement tools have a high degree of validity and reliability.

Validity reflects the measurement tool's ability to actually measure what it is supposed to. It also reflects how sensitive and specific the measurement is. Sensitivity reflects how well the test or tool identifies those with the disease, trait or condition. Specificity reflects how well the test or tool identifies those who do not have the disease, trait or condition.

Reliability refers to the measurement tool's ability to consistently measure the variable over time with the same results among the different data collectors. For example, an infection control professional who is exploring susceptibility to infection will want a valid measurement tool to measure "susceptibility", and not another variable, such as level of nutrition, age or any other factor that could possibly affect susceptibility.

Predictive values indicate how well the tool or test measurement is able to identify the number of people that have a positive test and also have the disease, trait or condition (positive predictive value) and how successfully the tool shows a negative test for those who are not affected by the disease, trait or condition (negative predictive value). Predictive values yield results that can be true positive, false positive, true negative and false negative.

The infection control professional will also consider the reliability of the measurement tool in terms of how the same, or similar, results occur regardless of the person collecting the data and regardless of when the data is collected. The results of the data collection must be consistent among data collectors and consistent across time. In summary, reliability reflects the accuracy and repeatability, or consistency, of the measure over time, regardless of who (inter-observer and intra-observer) performs the measurement.

Data for epidemiological study and research can come from a wide variety of sources including:

- Data regularly collected by other bodies and agencies, such as vital records statistics (birth and death rates) and CDC statistics

- Data collected by other reliable agencies for a purpose other than the research at hand, like data routinely collected by a state health department

- Data collected by the researcher (original data) for the purpose of the study

ANTIMICROBIALS

Antimicrobials can be classified as microbicidal and microbiostatics, and according to the specific type of microorganism that they act against. Microbicidal agents destroy microbes and microbiostatics inhibit growth and reproduction.

TYPES OF ANTIMICROBIALS

ANTIBACTERIAL DRUGS

Antibacterial drugs, commonly called antibiotics, are probably one of the most commonly used, and misused, type of medication.

Antibiotics	
Drug Classification	**Examples**
Aminoglycosides	Gentamicin, neomycin
Ansamycins	Streptomycin, Rifaximin
Carbapenems	Doripenem, Ettapenem
1st Gen Cephalosporins	Cefazolin, Cefalexin
2nd Gen Cephalosporins	Cefaclor, Cephoxitin
3rd Gen Cephalosporins	Ceifixime, Cefdinir
4th Gen Cephalosporins	Cefclidine, Cefepime
5th Gen Cephalosporins	Ceftobiprole, Ceftaroline Fosamil
Glycopeptides	Vancomycin, Telavancin
Lincosamides	Clindamysin, Lincomycin
Macrolides	Erythromycin, Spiramycin
Nitrofurans	Nitrofurantoin, Furazolidone
Penicillins	Ampicillin, Carbenicillin
Quinolones	Coprofloxacin, Levofloxacine
Sulfonamides	Silver Sulfadiazine, Mefenide
Tetracyclines	Tetracycline, Doxycycline

ANTIFUNGAL DRUGS

Antifungal drugs kill or prevent the growth of fungi. Some infections treated with these are thrush, athlete's foot and ringworm.

Antifungals	
Drug Classification	**Examples**
Polyene	Amphotericin, Nystatin
Azole	Fluconazole, Ketoconazole
Allylamine/Morpholine	Nafifine, Amorolfine
Antimetabolite	5-Fluorocytosine

ANTIVIRAL DRUGS

Antiviral drugs are used for specific viruses in the same manner that antibiotics are used for specific bacteria. They are commonly used for retroviruses like HIV, herpes, influenza and viral hepatitis. Examples include oseltamivir and acyclovir.

ANTIPARASITE DRUGS

Antiparasite medications are used to treat infections caused by parasitic cestodes, nematodes, protozoa and amoebae.

Antiparasitics	
Drug	**Condition Treated:**
Atovaquone-Proguanil	Malaria
Metronidazole, Tinidazole	Amebiasis, Giardiasis, Trichomoniasis
Ivermectin	Pinworms, Roundworms, Lice, Scabies
Pyrantel Pamoate	Enterobiasis, Hookworms
Albendazole	Tapeworm

USES OF ANTIMICROBIALS

THERAPEUTIC

The use of antimicrobials for the treatment of infections is the most common therapeutic treatment. To the greatest extent possible, the selection of the antimicrobial and the dosage should be driven by the specific microorganism and the current physical condition of the host.

Ideally, the therapeutic use of antimicrobials should be based on the components of the cycle of infection. For example, it should be based on the site of the infection, the host, and whenever possible, based on a definitive diagnosis of the infection and the offending pathogen. At times when there is not yet a definitive diagnosis, the empiric use of antimicrobials is indicated (we will cover empiric use later in this section.)

The identification of the specific offending pathogen is extremely important, especially when an infection can be life threatening, when the patient is not responding to current therapeutic interventions, and when the course of antimicrobial therapy may be prolonged.

Identification is dependent upon accurate and timely microbiological laboratory testing prior to the initiation of the therapy (when possible.) In addition to laboratory testing, the patient's medical history, including exposure history, and the presenting signs and symptoms also serve as considerations in terms of exactly which antimicrobial will be most effective and appropriate.

The initiation of antimicrobial therapy is based on a number of considerations including the condition of the patient. For example, critically ill patients, like those with sepsis, should have an immediate initiation of antimicrobial therapy immediately after diagnostic specimens are obtained. When the patient condition is stable, it is recommended that antimicrobial therapy be postponed until laboratory findings are complete.

PROPHYLACTIC

Antimicrobial prophylaxis can be a primary or secondary prevention measure. Primary prevents infection, and secondary treats/prevents recurrence.

Antimicrobial prophylaxis is often used to prevent the onset of an infectious disease. For example, preventive prophylactic antibiotics can be used for the prevention of urinary tract infections when a patient has an indwelling urinary catheter, and to prevent other infections such as rheumatic fever which can lead to serious cardiac damage, herpes simplex recurring bouts of cellulitis, meningitis, endocarditis, as well as open wound and open fracture infections.

Prophylactic antimicrobials, particularly anti-bacterials, are also used and indicated in a perioperative manner for certain types of surgery, like gastrointestinal and total joint replacement surgical procedures, to prevent surgically related infections. For example, an intravenous antibiotic may be administered ½ hour to 1 hour prior to a surgical procedure.

Ideally, prophylactic antimicrobials should be judiciously used only when necessary. The ideal prophylactic antimicrobial should be limited, inexpensive, nontoxic, target specific and bactericidal. Resistance remains a high public health concern.

EMPIRIC

The empiric use of antimicrobials is defined as the use of antimicrobial medications based on empiric signs and symptoms in the patient's physical condition, as contrasted with therapeutic use of antimicrobials, which are based on microbiological testing. Empiric use is indicated when a patient needs immediate treatment, and can't wait for laboratory results, which typically take 24 to 72 hours.

The antimicrobial agents used with empiric, rather than definitive, diagnoses are typically broad scope agents or a combination of agents that treat infection until a definitive diagnosis can be made.

ENVIRONMENTAL MONITORING

A biological environmental hazard is a health-related hazard in the environment that is infectious or biologically noxious in nature. Examples include contaminated water, contaminated food, infectious diseases, and bio-hazardous medical waste. Most biological environmental hazards affect people of all age groups. Age-specific biological environmental hazards include:

- *Infants and Young Children-* Infectious diseases, including childhood diseases that can often be prevented with immunizations, include prenatally acquired AIDS, gastrointestinal and respiratory illnesses that occur as the result of an immature immune system, poor hand washing and a tendency to put things, including dirty hands and fingers, in the mouth.

- *School Age Children-* Upper respiratory infections, such as influenza and strep throat, as a result of their close proximity to other children in the classroom and their tendency to have less than adequate hand washing practices. Other infections include otitis media, gastrointestinal infestations, pediculosis (lice) and scabies.

- *Adolescents-* A wide variety of sexually transmitted diseases (STDs) like hepatitis B, HIV, chlamydia, herpes simplex, Epstein-Barr virus (infectious mononucleosis) and meningococcal disease, particularly in college dormitories.

- *Young Adults and Middle-Aged Adults-* Sexually transmitted diseases, cervical cancer, biological risk factors in the workplace like exposures to blood, bodily fluids, and bio-hazardous wastes.

- *Older Adults-* Older adults, particularly those affected with an immune disorder and/or by diminished immune function associated with the normal aging process, are at risk for biological threats such as influenza, tuberculosis and pneumococcal infections.

SURVEILLANCE, ANALYSIS AND CHANGE

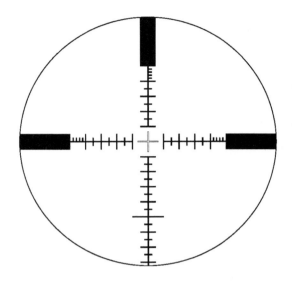

The information in this section will provide you with the knowledge, skills and abilities to conduct surveillance and epidemiologic investigations. You will learn about the design of surveillance systems, methods of data collection and compilation, and how to analyze and use surveillance data in your practice, in order to effect epidemiological change across the populations that you study and serve.

SURVEILLANCE

Public health surveillance is the methodical, ongoing and systematic collection, analysis, interpretation, and dissemination of data relating to a public health concern, including infectious diseases. The purpose of surveillance is to:

- Guide decision making
- Enable immediate action
- Determine/measure the impact of an event
- Identify populations at risk
- Identify the emergence of new threats
- Detect epidemics and pandemics
- Facilitate the establishment of priorities
- Provide an opportunity to research and investigate the course of specific health problems

- Help guide public policy
- Guide the planning, implementation and evaluation of a wide variety of initiatives to identify and control the spread of infection and other threats to public health.

SURVEILLANCE SYSTEM DESIGN

The design of a good surveillance system should include:

- Stakeholder involvement
- A description of the surveillance system
- The purpose of the surveillance system
- The operation of the surveillance system
- The dissemination of surveillance findings

STAKEHOLDER INVOLVEMENT

Stakeholders should be included in all phases of the surveillance process. Stakeholders include those individuals and groups who can use the efforts of the surveillance in terms of their health promotion and the prevention of disease. For example, on the community level, the stakeholders can include healthcare personnel from local hospitals and clinics; on the facility or corporate level, the stakeholders should include patients, family members and members of the specific facility.

DESCRIPTION

The description should include the importance of the system, the purpose of the system, the operation of the system and the resources that are needed to sustain and operate the system.

Some of the data that can be used to defend the importance of the surveillance system include the costs of not having one. For example, effective surveillance systems can:

- Decrease the frequency of an event
- Decrease the severity of an event
- Decrease the human and financial costs of events
- Prevent events
- Eliminate and/or decrease disparities and inequities associated with health promotion and illness prevention

Prevention and preventability is defined in terms of primary, secondary and tertiary prevention.

- Primary prevention prevents the occurrence of an event
- Secondary prevention is the early detection of an event and early interventions to stop, reverse or slow the progress/severity of the event
- Tertiary prevention aims to decrease, minimize or eliminate the complications and effects of the event after it has occurred.

PURPOSE

The surveillance system design should include a statement about its purpose and its objectives in addition to details about data collection, including the projected uses of collected data and the legal and regulatory authorities for data collection, such as the CDC, JCAHO or the state.

Other considerations include the system's relationship to other structures within the community or the organization, and the components of surveillance data collection activities. These components consist of:

- The population under surveillance

- The duration of the data collection
- The method of data collection
- The manner with which the data is managed and secured
- How the data is analyzed and disseminated
- The policies and procedures that ensure patient privacy, data confidentiality, and system security according to the federal government, the state government and other external regulatory bodies

OPERATION

When surveillance is indicated, the infection control professional should clearly define the event to the greatest level of specificity and refinement as possible. This definition can include several variables, including:

- Signs, symptoms and manifestations of the event
- Laboratory and other diagnostic test results
- People or population affected
- Place and time of event occurrence
- Some indication of certainty; for example, the event may be possible, suspected, probable, presumptive, definite or confirmed.

The steps of the surveillance process should also be determined and documented such as that shown in the diagram on the next page.

FIGURE 1. Simplified flow chart for a generic surveillance system

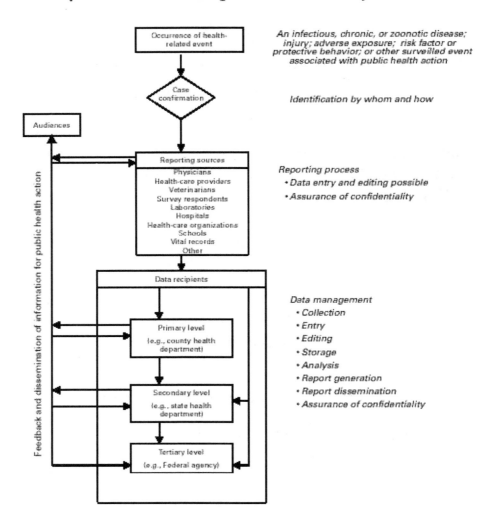

DISSEMINATING SURVEILLANCE FINDINGS

There are a variety of ways to disseminate the findings of surveillance activities. Some methods are widespread and formal, others are narrow and informal; still others can fall anywhere in the continuum from widespread to local and from formal to informal. Privacy and confidentiality must be maintained.

Some formal mechanisms for disseminating data include professional journal publications, presentations at national meetings and conferences and press releases. Less formal mechanism (also more geographically limited) are newsletters, community meetings, internal committee meetings, town hall meetings and bulletin or newsletter publications.

All reports must be understandable and usable by the target audience. For example, if you are presenting information about an influenza outbreak to a local community group of senior citizens, you will have to present the data and findings in terms that the group can understand. You will also need to address practical ways that they can protect themselves so that the information is usable and beneficial to their health.

PRIVACY

Data coding using standardized classifications, such as those put forward by the College of American Pathologists' Systematized Nomenclature of Medicine (CSTE), ensure some aspects of privacy and confidentiality of data. Security of data is also included in the regulations of HIPPA's Security Rule. The CDC and the National Modifiable Disease Surveillance System strive to ensure this confidentiality.

Some unique situations call for specific measures. For example, much data can be protected with the elimination of personal unique data and aggregation; however, when data is collected in an activity with a small sample size, or in case studies, it may be very difficult to protect the subjects' rights to privacy and confidentiality.

A related concern in protecting health data is data release, including procedures for releasing record-level, aggregate tabular and computer-based, interactive query systems data. The CDC and CSTE have negotiated a policy for the release of data from the National Modifiable Disease Surveillance System to facilitate use for public health while preserving the confidentiality of the data.

Records management, the acquisition of data and the disclosure of data must be consistent with the laws of privacy and security; it is a professional and legal responsibility.

SURVEILLANCE RESOURCES

Surveillance activities require resources. Costs associated with these systems are both direct and indirect. The system will need staff, financial resources, space, lighting, heat, supplies and equipment. At times, funding can be obtained through federal, state and local government or philanthropic grants.

SYSTEM EVALUATION

Evaluating a surveillance system can take many forms. Most processes include a determination of whether or not the purpose of the system is consistently upheld, the stakeholders and users of the data have their interests and needs met, and the entire system is consistent with legal and regulatory mandates.

Other considerations include usefulness, simplicity, flexibility, quality of the data, acceptability to others, sensitivity, predictive value, timeliness, responsiveness, stability and representativeness.

- **Usefulness** - Does the surveillance prevent and control infections? Is it able to detect infections, determine the degree of morbidity and mortality and prevent them?

- **Simplicity** - Can the system be easily and correctly used without excessive time and resources?

- **Flexibility** - Can the system adapt and respond to changing demands?

- **Acceptability** - Are people willing to participate in the system?

- **Sensitivity** - Can the system detect outbreaks and monitor changes in the number of cases over time?

- **Predictive Value** - Does the system accurately report cases related to the event without erroneous data and reports?

- **Representative** - Does the system correctly and accurately describe the event over time, and its distribution in the population by place and person, so the findings can be generalized to other populations?

- **Timeliness** - Can the system get the job done in time to prevent events?

- **Stability** - Are the system's immediate measures to detect and prevent events reliable and available?

No surveillance system is perfect, but all surveillance systems must be periodically evaluated in order to ensure that the system is working, particularly in light of the fact that surveillance is often costly.

HEPATITIS B AND HEPATITIS C SURVEILLANCE

One of the challenges associated with hepatitis surveillance is diagnosis, because quite often, the affected patient is asymptomatic and the duration of the exposure time to the onset of symptoms and confirmatory serological tests can be quite long. Acute hepatitis B may be from six weeks to six months and the duration for hepatitis C can range from two weeks to six months.

Hepatitis B is often symptomatic, but when these signs and symptoms appear they can include joint pain, fatigue, malaise, loss of appetite, nausea, vomiting, jaundice and dark urine. Serological tests indicative of acute hepatitis B include a positive hepatitis B IgM core antibody (IgM anti-HBc) AND a positive hepatitis B surface antigen (HBsAg).

Hepatitis C, unlike hepatitis B, has no serological tests that differentiate acute hepatitis C from chronic hepatitis C. It is, instead, the symptoms and signs that differentiate the chronic and acute forms. Acute hepatitis C is usually asymptomatic; the signs and symptoms of chronic hepatitis C include joint pain, fatigue, malaise, loss of appetite, nausea, vomiting, jaundice and dark urine.

INTEGRATING SURVEILLANCE ACTIVITIES INTO VARIOUS HEALTHCARE SETTINGS

According to sound professional judgment and the regulations of external regulatory bodies, surveillance activities must be integrated into all healthcare settings including acute care, long term care, home health care and ambulatory care settings.

The principles and the procedures relating to surveillance activities may have to be adapted and modified according to the setting and its population; however, it is expected that all healthcare settings have infection control and surveillance activities in place.

RESEARCH AND DATA

Research is classified in two ways: qualitative and quantitative. Quantitative research examines the relationship between independent and dependent, or outcome, variables. Qualitative research deeply analyzes non-numerical data, exploring meaning, values, experiences and achieving more in-depth understanding of a phenomenon of interest.

Research can further be categorized as descriptive and explanatory. For example, an infection control researcher must decide during the planning process whether they want to know *why* something is happening (explanatory) or whether they want to know *what* is happening (descriptive.)

QUANTITATIVE RESEARCH

Quantitative research is an empirical, systematic investigation of phenomena using statistical, mathematical techniques for data analysis. Quantitative research is more commonly used than qualitative research. The reason for the popularity of quantitative research is that many consider this method as "hard science" – that is, more scientific than qualitative research. Quantitative research studies are often more objective than qualitative studies, and the findings can be generalized.

Quantitative research involves the use of numbers, mathematics and statistics. It is a logical, deductive and systematic approach to research. The researcher manipulates the independent variable and they then observe and measure the changes and influences that result from the manipulation. Changes should occur in the dependent variable(s) when the independent variable is manipulated and/or an intervention is introduced. Quantitative research is deductive and qualitative research is inductive and more subject to subjectivity and discovery. Designs used for quantitative research include:

- Quasi-experimental design
- Meta-analysis
- Experimental design
- Non-experimental design
- Cross sectional design
- Longitudinal research
- Retrospective and prospective research

Quantitative research activities can be either experimental or descriptive. A descriptive research study measures the dependent variable once and an experimental research study has both pre-intervention measurement and post-intervention measures. Subjects are measured before and after a treatment.

VARIABLES

There are three basic types of variables: independent, dependent and extraneous.

An *independent variable* is the factor that has some influence on the dependent variable, or variables. Independent variables can be manipulated in order to determine the relationship between these changes and changes in the dependent variable.

A *dependent variable* is the factor that changes as a result of the influence of the independent variable. It is the behavior, outcome or characteristic that the researcher hopes to predict or explain. A dependent variable changes as a response to some manipulation. For this reason, a dependent variable is sometimes referred to as a response variable.

When one is researching infection rates among critical care patients, data regarding infections (dependent or response variable) will be influenced by the independent variable (the critical status of the patient).

Extraneous variables, also called interfering variables, are conditions or phenomenon that undesirably impact on the dependent variable. Valid research findings are threatened because of these interfering variables so they must be eliminated, or at least controlled.

MEASUREMENT AND BIAS

The process of measurement is central to quantitative research. Measurement provides the basic, fundamental connection between empirical observation and a mathematical expression of quantitative relationships. For example, we are able to measure certain things like blood pressure and pulse rates using equipment (blood pressure) and tactile senses (pulse rate). There are, however, many things that we cannot measure directly with our empirical senses and equipment. For example, we cannot easily measure variables like pain, fear, comfort, anxiety, satisfaction and similar concepts using equipment or the empirical senses. Measurement tools are developed to attempt to measure, and quantify, these non-empirical variables.

Bias is usually not conscious – it can be reduced in quantitative research by performing "double blind" studies. This means using an adequate sample size, and randomly assigning subjects to the experimental and control groups while ensuring that both the subjects and researcher are "blind" to the experimental treatments.

The characteristics of the subjects are also important in quantitative research. It is suggested that a relatively homogenous, or similar, group of subjects be included in the study so that the effects of the experimental intervention are more like to occur as the result of the intervention, rather than some varying characteristic intrinsic to the subjects.

TYPES OF DATA

There are two types of data: quantitative and qualitative.

Quantitative data is numerical. It is analyzed with mathematics, including statistics.

Qualitative data, on the other hand, is narrative. It consists of the identification of patterns, trends and themes found in data which is most often obtained using focus group or interview techniques.

GENERATING DATA

Data generation is essentially collecting data regarding the variables that are going to be studied. For example, if you are exploring the relationship between lengths of stay and infection rates, you will have to collect data about lengths of stay and infection rates.

Physiological, psychological and social variables are the most commonly occurring variables that healthcare professional's research. An example of a physiological variable is a white blood cell count. Examples of psychological variables include things like anxiety, depression and level of orientation. An example of a social variable is the level of interaction among patients and infection control nurses, or other infection control staff.

SCALES

A scale is a measurement instrument, or tool, that is used for the collection of quantitative data. There are several types of scales, including:

- Likert type scales
- Guttman scales
- Multiple choice scales
- Yes-No scales

Likert Scales

Likert scales are highly useful and perhaps the most commonly used type of scale in research and other investigational studies. The Likert (or Likert type) scale measures how strongly a person agrees or disagrees with a specific statement. A Likert scale, for example, can measure how strongly a patient agrees or disagree with a statement like, "I believe that the infection control professionals met my needs."

This will be measured on a scale similar to the one below:

1	2	3	4	5
Strongly Disagree	Disagree	Neutral	Agree	Strongly Agree

A typical Likert scale may have as many as twenty to thirty statements, or items, that the patient rates. The data obtained from a Likert scale can be analyzed using measures of central tendency like means, modes, and medians, as well as more complex statistics tools like standard deviation.

Guttman Scales

A Guttman scale is a comparative scaling technique based on the premise that data can be collected along a continuum, and be ranked in order from the least extreme opinion to the most extreme opinion. One disadvantage of the Guttman scale is that it takes a lot of time, effort and skill to develop one. Here is an example of a Guttman scale item relating to infection control:

"All patients that have never been previously hospitalized should undergo infection control screening."

"All patients that are hospitalized should undergo infection control screening."

"All patients, regardless of hospitalization status, should undergo infection control screening."

Multiple Choice Scales

Multiple choice scales, like a multiple choice test, provide a fixed set of answers to choose from. These scales are useful for collecting factual information and are relatively quick and easy for subjects to respond to, unlike the Guttman scale, which often requires more thought. A disadvantage of this type of scale is that the developer of the scale may forget to include an important choice in these questions, and all items must be clear and free of any ambiguity. Here is an example of a multiple choice scale:

---

1. **What is your level of education?**

    _____ Less than a high school diploma

    _____ High school diploma

    _____ Associate's Degree

    _____ Bachelor's Degree

    _____ Graduate Degree

Yes or No Scales

Yes or no scales lend themselves to simple dichotomous data, but they do not produce rich, in-depth data that other scales can, such as the Likert scale.

DATA COLLECTION TECHNIQUES

There are many different data collection techniques. Some are relatively easy and cost effective and others are more difficult, challenging and costly. Additionally, some methods of data collection are suitable only for qualitative research and others are suitable for quantitative research.

Some of the considerations that an infection control professional use in planning a particular data collection method, or technique, include costs, the amount of time necessary to collect the data, the purpose and the setting of the investigation, needed resources and the characteristics of the subject or patients. Data collection techniques include:

- Questionnaires (Mailed and Telephonic)
- Focus Groups
- Diaries and Journals
- Observation
- Face-to-Face Interviews
- Logs
- Documents
- Critical Incidents
- Audits

QUESTIONNAIRES

Questionnaires are only as good as the people that construct them. The most commonly occurring questionnaire items, or questions, are closed- and open-ended questions. Closed-ended questions are easier for the questionnaire respondent to answer; a check mark or an X is often the only thing the responder has to do in order to answer closed yes or no questions. With open-ended questions, the responder has to compose and formulate their own response. For example, the subject may be asked to list at least three factors which they believe affect their state of health or wellness.

Questionnaires can be used as a primary data collection method, as well as in addition to other data collection methods. Self-completed questionnaires can also help to successfully avoid possible biases that occur with the interview process. Another advantage is that questionnaires can collect data from large population samples in a relatively short time, but the return rate with mailed questionnaires is often highly disappointing to the investigator.

Telephone questionnaires are a popular method particularly when public opinion polling is being done. Like a mailed questionnaire, a telephone questionnaire is a systematic collection of data from a sample population, but response rates are much higher and researchers have better control over the quality of the data without introducing bias.

FOCUS GROUPS

Focus group research is a relative newcomer to investigations and research in healthcare, but they have been used in the worlds of business and politics for decades. Focus groups can provide qualitative or quantitative data.

The first step of focus group research is the composition of an interview guide. This pre-planned interview guide should be done in collaboration with the stakeholders. The next step of focus group research is to select and invite the subjects to attend the focus group session; unlike other research methods, focus groups have a small number of subjects, or patients, in the sample. The groups usually have from six to ten participants in each group; questions are primarily open-ended.

During open discussion, the members of the focus group are free to interact with and respond to the ideas and thoughts of other participants. No value judgments are made during the discussions, and there are no correct or incorrect answers to the interview questions; all responses are good data that can, and should be, collected.

The data from focus group research is also not analyzed with statistical methods, but instead by reading and studying the narrative content for themes, patterns and trends.

DIARIES, JOURNALS AND LOGS

Diaries and journals, like focus groups, provide narrative data. The difference is that diaries and journals have written data and focus group data is oral. Similar to focus groups, diaries and journals can collect rich, qualitative data.

Researchers often use logs for less extensive data that tends to be quantitative, rather than qualitative. This usually differentiates logs from diaries and journals.

OBSERVATION

Observation is used to gather empirical data with the use of one's senses, such as sight, hearing, smell, and tactile sensations. Observation is a deliberate, conscious, objective process. The primary aspects of observation data collection are noticing and observing the data, selecting, organizing and interpreting the data.

An example of the observational technique of data collection is when the investigator observes that the patient's face is red and warm to the touch, while considering other variables such as the patient's temperature, the environmental temperature and the patient's level of activity when they are observing a flushed face. During this process, it is important to determine whether or not observational data is meaningful and significant.

There are some conditions that must be met in order for an observation to be considered scientific. These conditions are as follows:

- All observations must be controlled, unbiased, validated and checked

- The investigation's specific objectives must be consistent with the observations that are being performed

- The observations, collection of data and the recording of the observational data must be done according to a systematic plan

The four basic classifications of observation are concealment with intervention, concealment without intervention, no concealment with intervention and no concealment without intervention. Concealment refers to whether or not the subject knows that they are being observed; and intervention refers to whether or not the observer acts in a way that the leads to a change in the subject or patient. An example of concealment without intervention is the use of a one-way mirror to observe pediatric subjects engaging in parallel play.

Observational methods may be structured or unstructured. The use of structured observations is planned in terms of what behavior or events will be observed. This form of observation often uses pre-planned standardized tools, checklists and rating scales. Unstructured observational methods usually involve collecting descriptive information about the topic of interest; with this method, the observer keeps notes that record activities, as well as the interpretations of these activities during these observations.

Regardless of the method, objectivity and reliability among observers must be ensured.

Observation may be the only way for the researcher to study variables of interest. For example, self-reports (what people say they do) often don't match up with actual behavior. In this instance, the only way for the researcher to ensure the validity of their findings is to actually observe the subject and collect data based on the patient or subject behavior. Observations can be used in experimental, non-experimental designs and for field studies. This data is quite flexible for a wide variety of research studies and investigations.

FACE-TO-FACE INTERVIEWS

An interview is a form of oral communication with a purpose and plan. In the context of healthcare studies and investigations, the collection of data and the identification of potential problems are frequent reasons for using the interview research technique. This technique is also beneficial when clarification is needed, something that cannot be done, for example, when a questionnaire is mailed out.

The two approaches to interviewing are informal, or non-directive, and formal, which is directive and focused. Informal or non-directive interviews allow the patient, or patient, to control the pacing and the subject matter; with a formal interview, the control of the interview is with the interviewer, using a set of pre-planned questions with very little free discussion and flexibility.

The two types of interview questions are open- and closed-ended questions. Open ended questions facilitate meaningful, rich and full responses in terms of the patient's own beliefs, knowledge and feelings. Open ended questions usually begin with such words as "How", Why" or "Tell me about....." In sharp contrast, a closed ended question elicits only a "yes" or "no" or another single word answer. An example of an open-ended question is, "Tell me about your pain." An example of a closed-ended question is, "Do you believe that you have access to immunization resources?"

The personal interview method has both advantages and disadvantages. The advantages of this method of data collection are that interviews are often flexible and highly beneficial when you want detailed and in depth responses. The disadvantages of the face to face interview include the fact that they are time consuming, relatively costly and not appropriate for making generalizations. All forms of interview questions must be clear and free of any suggestion or bias.

DOCUMENTS

In healthcare, there are many different sources that can be used for obtaining document data and analysis. A researcher exploring whether or not a specific risk factor (other than one already known) affects infection, for example, may use documents such as journals, previous studies and patient medical records to uncover patterns relating to the health care concern or the phenomenon of interest.

CRITICAL INCIDENTS

Critical incident data can be collected to solve both practical problems and to develop broad principles and concepts. There are several ways to gather critical incident data and information, but in most cases, the subject is usually asked to describe an experience they have had. Critical incidents can be used in a variety of settings to explore many different situations and interactions. Critical incidents can be used to:

- Identify and resolve issues or problems
- Fact find
- Evaluate whether or not a particular solution has corrected problems and issues

AUDITS

The audit process entails the systematic review of care, or an aspect of care, compared to an established expectation of criteria. For this reason, the method is primarily used to review and study structures and processes, rather than outcomes – the overall goal is to collect data and review it in order to ensure that everyone is doing everything they're supposed to. Audits give data that can be used for corrective actions and planned change, but they are limited in terms of revealing intervention quality.

CROSS SECTIONAL, COHORT AND CASE CONTROL STUDIES

Longitudinal research studies the same group of individuals over an extended period of time and, at times, this research can last for decades. This research allows us to look at changes over time. There are three major types of longitudinal studies: Panel studies with a cross section of subjects, cohort studies and case control studies.

CROSS SECTIONAL PANEL STUDIES

Cross sectional panel studies collect information from the subjects relating to their disease and exposure status. They are useful for exploring the relationship between a variable and a disease, and not for determining cause and effect, which requires data over time. Case control and cohort studies are more capable of determining causality.

COHORT STUDIES

In cohort studies, the subjects have been exposed to the pathogen regardless of whether or not they have the infectious disease being studied. These studies are prospective, rather than retrospective, and they determine outcomes, then compare those outcomes to the individual's exposure. For example, a cohort study would examine individuals exposed to salmonella in a particular restaurant, interview them about their exposure in terms of the foods they ate, and then follow them over time to see if they develop complications.

Cohort studies have several advantages, including their ability to study multiple outcomes resulting from a single exposure, and their usefulness in studying rare exposures. Disadvantages include the costs and resources needed to conduct these types of studies, and the loss of subjects over time.

CASE CONTROL STUDIES

Case control studies work backwards from the effect to the suspected cause. Some of the advantages of case control studies are the ability to explore multiple exposures relating to a single outcome, their ability to study rare diseases and those with a prolonged latency period, and their relatively low cost. Disadvantages include the fact that they are not appropriate for rare exposures.

ORGANIZING DATA

Quantitative data is analyzed using one or more types of statistics. Generally, statistics can be described as descriptive and inferential.

The purpose of descriptive statistics is to organize and analyze large amounts of data in order to get some perspective or context. There are two basic types of descriptive statistics- measures of central tendency and measures of variability.

Measures of central tendency place numerical data near the middle, or center, of the "bell shaped curve". Numbers that cluster around the "middle" of a set of values are measures of central tendency. These middle numbers are called the mean, median and mode. The mean is the average of all of the values, or numbers, in a given numerical set. The *median* is the middle number in the sequence of numbers; the *mode* is the most frequently occurring number, or score, in the sequence of numbers or values.

FINDING THE MEAN

The mean is calculated by adding the values of all the numbers in the set, and then dividing this sum by the number of values included in the set. Here is an example:

$$[16, 24, 33, 76, 32, 17]$$

1. First, count the number of values in the set:

   [16   24   33   76   32   17]
     1   2   3   4   5   6

   There are six total values. This is the *divider*.

2. Now, add the values together:

   $$16 + 24 + 33 + 76 + 32 + 17 = 198$$

   198 is the *sum* of all the values.

3. Now, divide the *sum* by the *divider*.

   $$198 / 6 = 33$$

The mean, or average, of the set is 33.

The mean only tells us a small part of the entire picture. Other statistics are needed to fully understand the meaning of any measurement.

FINDING THE MEDIAN

The best way to determine the median, or the middle measurement, is by putting the numbers in either ascending or descending order and then finding the number or value that is in the middle of all the numbers or values. The determination of the median is not mathematical or statistical; however, it is still referred to as a statistical measure of central tendency.

Finding the median is slightly different when dealing with odd-numbered or even-numbered sets.

Finding the Median of an Odd-Numbered Set

"#$%&'(%&))%&†$%&)'

1. First, arrange the values in ascending order:

    &"#$&#*&   '(&   )'&   ))+& &   &&

    Lowest ⟶ Highest

2. Now, find the number in the middle of the set.

    "#$& #*& | 2¢& |)'&   ))+& &   &

The median of the set is 24.

Finding the Median of an Even-Numbered Set

1. First, arrange the values in ascending order:

    Lowest ⟶ Highest

2. Find the *pair of numbers* in the middle of the set:

    24 and 32 are the pair of numbers in the middle of the set.

3. Add the pair of numbers together:

    56 is the sum of the pair of numbers.

4. Divide the sum by two:

The median of the set is 28.

FINDING THE MODE

The mode is the value that occurs most often in a set of numbers. In determining the mode, it is often helpful to list the numbers in ascending or descending order, as with the median.

1. First, arrange the values in ascending order:

   Lowest ⟶ Highest

2. Find the number that occurs most often in the set:

   ... 32 32 ...

The mode of the set is 32.

Finding Bi-Modal Distribution

A set can have two modes – this is known as a bi-modal distribution.

1. First, arrange the values in ascending order:

   Lowest ──────────────▶ Highest

2. Find the numbers that occur most often in the set:

The two modes of this set are 16 and 32.

PRACTICAL APPLICATION

When all three measures of central tendency (mean, median and mode) in a set are the same, it's called "normal" distribution. However, normal distribution is pretty rare in real world statistics!

These measures of central tendency are often close, but not exactly the same, in research data. The mean and the median are the most commonly reported measures of central tendency; the mode is less often used.

The mean's disadvantages include the fact that it can be highly sensitive to extreme scores at the lower or higher end of the ordered set of numbers. The median is not as sensitive to extremes as the mean.

VARIABILITY

You already know that normal distribution is a fairly rare occurrence. Most of the time, the distribution is not normal – that is, the measurements of central tendency are different due to something called *variability*.

Measurements of variability include the range, variance and standard deviation.

The *range* indicates the largest and smallest of all the values. For example, using the set of values below, the range is from 18 (the smallest or lowest value) to 66 (the largest or greatest value). This value can be stated as "The range is from 18 to 66" or "The range is 48 (the difference between 66 and 18).

Variance is a useful statistical calculation that reflects how much the values vary around the mean. It is a measure that tells us how far apart the numbers are spread in the set, and how far the numbers are away from the mean. Simply stated, the variance is the average squared deviation of values away from the mean. Variance is symbolized by S^2.

The *standard deviation* is similar to variance in that it, too, shows how much variance or dispersion there is around the mean. A high standard deviation indicates that the data is spread out greatly around the mean; a low standard deviation indicates that the data is more closely aligned around the mean. The method of calculation for the standard deviation is to find the square root of the variance. Standard deviation is symbolized as S.

INFERENTIAL STATISTICS

Inferential statistics are far more complicated than descriptive measurements of central tendency and variance. Inferential statistics infer conclusions about the subjects of the study. They allow researchers to make predictions and generalize the results of a study to a larger population, provided that the sample was representative of the larger group or population.

CORRELATION DOES NOT IMPLY CAUSATION

It is virtually impossible to prove causality in research, because one can never be sure that they controlled for every possible variable in a test. In fact, one of the most important rules in all of science is the maxim, "Correlation does not imply causation."

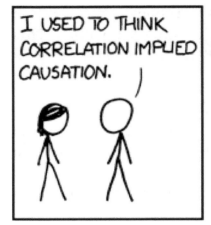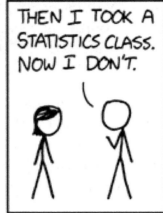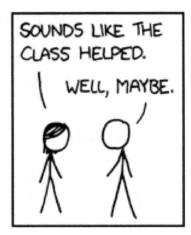

For example, let's say a researcher is comparing two studies of a given population – one measuring umbrella sales and one measuring average body weight. The researcher notices that when umbrella sales go up, so does average body weight. There is a correlation here – so does that mean that buying an umbrella could put people at greater risk of obesity?

Of course, this is silly - the most likely explanation is that when people buy umbrellas, it's late autumn or early winter, so they are spending less time outside being active, and enjoying holiday foods. The uptick in both umbrella sales and average body weight are a coincidence.

---

[5]Credit: Randall Munroe. Original: http://xkcd.com/552/ Used under license: http://creativecommons.org/licenses/by-nc/4.0/

USING CORRELATION COEFFICIENTS

Since it's almost impossible to prove causality with 100% accuracy (especially with human subjects) scientists use something called *correlation coefficients*.

There are two types of correlation: Positive and negative. A positive correlation occurs when both the independent and dependent variables increase or decrease. A negative correlation occurs when one of the variables increases and the other decreases.

Some examples of positive correlations are:

- The incidence of influenza decreases with population size (both decrease)
- The incidence of influenza increases with age (both increase)

Some examples of negative correlation include:

- Operative infection rates decrease when surveillance increases
- Operative infection rates increase when recovery room staff decreases

Some other inferential statistics are:

- Analysis of variance (ANOVA)
- Analysis of covariance (ANCOVA)
- Linear regression
- Regression analysis
- Factor analysis

STATISTICAL ERRORS

In the research context, an error is NOT a careless mistake, but an error that occurs despite careful and accurate calculations. There are two types of errors.

- *Type I-* This error occurs when a null hypothesis (the belief that two variables are unrelated) is false, but is accidentally accepted as fact. Also known as "false positive."

- *Type II-* This error occurs when a null hypothesis is accidentally rejected. Also known as "false negative."

A Type I error can lead one to conclude that a relationship exists between two events, when in fact there is no connection whatsoever (for instance, believing that buying an umbrella causes obesity.) False positives are a very common error in scientific research and statistical analysis.

A Type II error can lead a researcher to conclude that there were no differences in the dependent variable when indeed there was.

STATISTICAL SIGNIFICANCE

The T test and Chi square test tell us if the findings are, or are not, statistically significant. Simply stated, they tell us if results occurred as the result of chance, accident, or manipulation of the independent variable.

For example, when the result of a T test is $p < .05$, it means that there is a less than a 5 % possibility that an accident has occurred. The results are primarily related to the research itself, at about 95%. $p < .20$ means that random chance accounts for less than 20%, and about 80% of the change is related to the manipulation of the independent variable rather than chance or accident.

The consideration of chance is very important when it comes to human subjects. When, for example, a pharmaceutical study is investigating the life-threatening side effects of a new medication and the study indicates p < .20, you would not want to generalize these findings to others, because 20% of the findings are related to chance and *not* the study itself.

In other studies, like nursing research studies without any risks, a p < .05 or p < .10 can be tolerated. With life-threatening studies a p < .01 or less is typically acceptable.

ANALYZING DATA

QUALITATIVE DATA

The analysis of qualitative data is quite different from the analysis of quantitative data; it is narrative and not numerical. Qualitative data are carefully analyzed for patterns, trends and themes, instead of statistics or math.

The process of analysis for qualitative studies can be a lengthy and tedious process. All data is read word by word and the researcher critically thinks about the data and then they organize it into categories, themes, patterns, content and key points. The data is analyzed using inductive thinking and logic rather than deductive reasoning. You have moved from a general concept like medication compliance to specifics such as family support.

QUANTITATIVE DATA

Quantitative data is analyzed by using one or more types of statistics. Generally, statistics can be described as descriptive and inferential statistics. Various statistical methods and calculations were fully discussed above.

Not too long ago, researchers had to calculate statistics using only a paper and pencil. Now, there is a wide variety of statistical software programs that not only ensure greater accuracy, but also make it unnecessary to have to compute complex equations. In the modern era, it is more important to understand what a specific statistic means and how to interpret the results in research, rather than performing complex mathematic procedures.

BENCHMARKING

When an infection control practitioner has completed a surveillance study, they will want to know how their results compare to others. Are their infection rates lower? Is the incidence of postoperative infections greater? Is their incidence of postoperative infections rarer with their best practices, rather than others'?

In order to find the answers to these questions, the researchers use a tool called *benchmarking*. The 12 phases of the benchmarking process are:

1. Select the subject
2. Define the process under study
3. Identify potential partners like other hospitals
4. Identify data sources like professional journals and published benchmarks
5. Collect data and select partners
6. Determine the gap
7. Establish process differences
8. Target future performance
9. Communicate
10. Adjust the goal as needed
11. Implement a correct action or planned change
12. Review and recalibrate

Benchmarking is categorized as either internal or external.

Internal benchmarking compares the performance of two or more different groups in the same organization. For example, an infection control professional may want to compare the number of hospital-acquired infections among different nursing care units in the medical center.

External benchmarking compares the performance of your healthcare agency with two or more different groups outside of the organization.

Benchmarking can also be classified and categorized as process, performance, operational and strategic benchmarking.

INTERPRETING ANTIBIOTIC RESISTANCE PATTERNS

The National Antimicrobial Resistance Monitoring System for Enteric Bacteria (NARMS), in collaboration with the CDC, state and local public health departments, the US Food and Drug Administration and the US Department of Agriculture, survey and track all changes in the antimicrobial susceptibility of certain enteric bacteria, food animals and meats in order to protect public health. This surveillance identifies patterns of emerging resistance to protect people from resistant infections, which are one of the nation's most serious health threats.

Some ways that these resistant strains can be prevented are the careful and judicious use of antibiotics, adhering to food safety, preventing infections from occurring, preventing resistant bacteria from spreading, tracking resistant bacteria and promoting the development of new antibiotics and new diagnostic tests for resistant bacteria.

The CDC conducts antibiotic susceptibility using isolates from both outbreaks and isolated, sporadic cases of infection. Some of the sporadic infections that the CDC tests include salmonella, shigella, E. coli, Campylobacter and the vibrio species except V. cholerae. Outbreak studies allow the CDC to identify and more fully understand the source of the outbreak.

CLASSIFICATIONS OF ANTIBIOTIC-RESISTANT BACTERIA

Urgent Threat

- Clostridium difficile
- Carbapenem-resistant Enterobacteriaceae (CRE)
- Drug-resistant Neisseria gonorrhoeae

Serious Threat

- Multidrug-resistant Acinetobacter
- Drug-resistant Campylobacter

- Fluconazole-resistant Candida
- Extended spectrum β-lactamase producing Enterobacteriaceae (ESBLs)
- Vancomycin-resistant Enterococcus
- Multidrug-resistant Pseudomonas aeruginosa
- Drug-resistant Non-typhoidal Salmonella
- Drug-resistant Salmonella Typhi
- Drug-resistant Shigella
- Methicillin-resistant Staphylococcus aureus (MRSA)
- Drug-resistant Streptococcus pneumoniae
- Drug-resistant tuberculosis

Concerning Threat

- *Vancomycin-resistant Staphylococcus aureus (VRSA)*
- *Erythromycin-resistant Group A Streptococcus*
- *Clindamycin-resistant Group B Streptococcus*

PREPARING INVESTIGATION REPORTS

The findings of epidemiologic investigations must logically relate and interpret the findings of the study.

CONCLUSIONS, IMPLICATIONS, LIMITATIONS AND RECOMMENDATIONS

Conclusions include summarizing statements that relate to the data. The implications typically relate to why the study was an important one and how the study can be used by others for practice changes or further research.

The limitations of the study include statements about why the results may not, or should not, be immediately used and/or applied to different populations. The recommendations of the study include things like suggested ideas for future study.

INCLUDING TABLES, GRAPHS AND CHARTS

Tables, charts and graphs are a great way to display data in surveillance reports and during group processes such as performance improvement activities. Some of the most commonly used tables, graphs and charts are:

- Cause-and-effect diagrams, such as "fishbone" or Ishikawa diagrams
- Check sheets
- Control charts
- Histograms
- Pareto charts
- Scatter diagrams
- Stratification charts, also referred to as a flow chart or a run chart
- PIE charts
- Bar graphs
- Line graphs

COMMUNICATING RESEARCH RESULTS

The last step of the research process is communicating results. This is often neglected but it is highly important, particularly when you consider the fact that research should improve healthcare and healthcare practice.

RATES

A rate is the mathematical measure of the frequency of the disease or health care problem in a specified period of time. In this chapter, you'll find a brief explanation of the key concepts related to rates.

RATIO

The mathematical relationship between two numbers; for example, if the rate of hospital acquired infections occur in 1 of every 1,000 inpatients and 1 in 5,000 outpatients, these ratios can be expressed as 1:1,000 and 1:5,000, respectively.

INCIDENCE

Incidence is the number of newly diagnosed cases in a specific population during a defined period of time. This rate is calculated by dividing the number of new cases by the number of people in the risk population. For example, the incidence of black lung disease among coal miners may be 250 per 10,000 or 2.5%.

PREVALENCE

Prevalence is an epidemiological statistic that measures how widespread a disease is at a particular time. A prevalence rate is expressed in proportion with the numerator as the number of people with the disease and the denominator as the total number of people who may or may not be at risk for the disease. For example, if there are 100 people in a long term care facility and 30 of these residents now have pneumonia, the prevalence is 30%.

CRUDE/ADJUSTED RATES

Rates can sometimes be expressed as a crude rate or an adjusted rate. A crude rate is simply the number of cases in a population at a specified period of time; and an adjusted rate gives more information about the number of cases by placing it within the context of a subpopulation or subgroup like a job category or an age group.

Rates are adjusted using a mathematical direct or indirect adjustment. A direct adjustment is used when the rate for the specific population is known; and an indirect adjustment is used when the rate is not known.

INCIDENCE RATE

An incidence rate represents the number of new events, which is mathematically calculated by dividing the number of new events by the number of people in the risk population and expressing the incidence rate per 1,000 or 10,000 people or as a percentage.

INCIDENCE PROPORTION

An incidence proportion is the proportion of a population affected by a particular disease, like an infectious disease, or another medical disorder during a specified period of time.

MORTALITY RATES

Mortality rates can be expressed and reported as an adjusted rate that accommodates for population characteristics such as age and as a crude rate without any contextual adjustments. Commonly used and cited mortality rates are varied. Some mortality rates are:

- *Infant Mortality Rates-* An infant mortality rate reflects the mathematical number of babies less than one year of age who have died over the total number of live infants born during that year.

- *Neonatal Mortality Rates-* Neonatal mortality rates are the number of newborns who are less than 28 days old over the total number of live infants born during that year.

- *Post-neonatal Mortality Rates-* Post-neonatal mortality rates, similar to neonatal mortality rates, are the number of newborns from 28 days of age to one year of age over the total number of live infants born during that year.

- *Age Specific Mortality Rates-* Similar to infant mortality rates, age specific mortality rates are calculated for age groups such as toddlers, preschool children, school age children, adolescents, young adults, middle year adults and the elderly.

- *Cause Specific Mortality Rates-* Cause specific mortality rates represent the number of deaths from a specific cause divided by the number of people in the population. For example, a cause specific mortality rate can be calculated to communicate the number of deaths related to pneumonia within a particular population like males, females, and hospitalized elders.

- *Proportionate Mortality Rates-* A proportionate mortality rate is a mathematical ratio that reflects the number of deaths attributable to a specific cause over the total number of deaths during a specific period of time.

- *Case Fatality Rates-* Case fatality rates reflect of the number of deaths that have occurred among those with a specific disease or disorder. Mathematically, it is the number of deaths divided by the number affected by the specified disease, such as an infectious illness.

MORBIDITY RATES

Morbidity rates tell us about the rates of illness, diseases, infections, disability etc. Morbidity can be discussed in terms of prevalence, incidence and survival rates, among other ways.

- *Attack Rates* - Attack rates reflect the proportion of people who have been exposed to an agent and who have also developed the disease. For example, an attack rate may describe the number of people who have gotten ill after drinking contaminated water or ingesting infected, contaminated food.

- *Survival Rates* - Survival rates describe the rates of survival among a group or population that is affected with a health related event like an infection.

CALCULATING INFECTION RATES

Knowing infection rates can be useful in terms of prevention when the rates are specific to a provider, care unit, device or procedure. For example, surveillance data, when aggregated over time, may reveal a number of usable conclusions, including the fact that one or more providers are associated with hospital-acquired infections. Surveillance data may also reveal that one unit, or patient care area, has more hospital-acquired infections than other units.

Similarly, certain devices like endoscopy equipment, may also have a greater than expected infection rate, and some procedures like endoscopy or orthopedic surgery may have a greater than expected prevalence of infection.

After data is collected and analyzed to reveal these types of specific infections, the infection control professional must determine why this is occurring. For example, a particular nursing care unit may need some continuing education on correct hand washing procedures or there may be a deficient piece of sterilizing equipment outside an operating room.

INCORPORATING FINDINGS INTO RATE CALCULATIONS

Calculating and determining infections and infection rates after discharge is a challenging but highly important part of infection control activities. For example, postoperative infections must be explored during the course of hospitalization, but also after the patient has been discharged. Some challenges associated with this type of surveillance include the fact that surgical infections, for example, can occur up to a month after surgery. Other challenges are associated with a number of variables outside of the healthcare environment over which the healthcare facility has little control over. For example, if a wound infection occurs, it is often difficult to determine if the infection was the result of poor wound care by the patient, an unsanitary home environment or exposure to infections in the community.

RISK

Risk is a function of several forces, including exposure potential and susceptibility. Simply defined, risk is the probability or likelihood that a disease will occur. An individual, family, group or population is at risk when they, more than others, are susceptible to disease.

Some patients (individuals, families, groups and/or populations are at greater risk than other patients because they have been exposed more than others. For example, oncology nurses are at greater risk for the hazards associated with contaminated sharps than other groups, or populations, because they have a greater exposure risk.

Some patients are at greater risk than others because they are more susceptible than others. For example, some patients are more susceptible to diseases and disorders because they are vulnerable and they lack natural defenses, as is the case with opportunistic infections among HIV/AIDS patients. Another example is the risk for cancer as based on some genetic factor(s) that places a person at risk for cancer.

Populations at risk, referred to as target groups, are targeted for interventions because they have been identified as "at risk".

One way of conceptualizing risk and risk factors among individuals and groups is by applying the Seven Components of Wellness, plus cultural factors, as shown below:

- *Physical Risk Factors-* Genetics, poor nutrition, the lack of regular exercise, age, obesity, poor lifestyle choices, risky behaviors, such as illicit drugs and unprotected sex, disability, and the presence of an illness or infection are examples of physical or biological risk factors.

- *Social and Economic Risk Factors-*Some social and economic risk factors include a lack of relationships with others, including intimate relationships, a lack of social support, poverty, homelessness, and the lack of access to available and affordable healthcare resources

- *Emotional and Psychological Risk Factors-* Stress, ineffective coping skills, depression, the lack of insight, emotional distress, physiological defense mechanisms like denial, and one's lack of acceptance of one's own limitations are examples of emotional and psychological risk factors that can impact on one's illness. There is a strong mind-body interaction.

- *Intellectual Risk Factors-* Cognitive limitations, decreased levels of consciousness, literacy, and level of education impact on the occurrence of illness and disease. For example, some patients do not utilize preventive care services because they do not understand the benefits of it.

- *Spiritual Risk Factors-* A patient who perceives that they do not have a purpose in life and/or find no meaning or fullness in life is more prone to illness than others.

- *Occupational Risk Factors-* Some occupations are filled with risk and others are not. For example, people who cut trees, roofers, miners, heavy equipment operators, and those exposed to environmental toxins, such as asbestos and chemicals are at greater risk for illness, accidents and disease because of the very nature of their job or occupation. People with office jobs are at least risk. Avocations, or hobbies, like sky diving and mountain climbing can also increase the patient's risk of disease, accidents, and illness.

- *Environmental Risk Factors-* Poor air and water, the lack of adequate and safe food, as well as failures to provide basic safety measures in the environment also place patients and populations at risk.

- *Cultural Risk Factors-* Some examples of cultural risk factors include unhealthy dietary practices and traditions, ritualistic scarring and health related beliefs and practices, like using the services of a medicine man rather than a physician, place risk on the patient as a result of their cultural beliefs and practices.

RELATED CONCEPTS

Some of the concepts relating to risk include:

- Susceptibility
- Exposure potential
- Relative risk ratios

Risk can be defined as the likelihood, or probability, that an event, such as a disease, will occur. Risk and risk factors indicate that an individual or group is more susceptible to an event than others. For example, an individual may be at risk for a sexually transmitted disease, and much more susceptible than others, because they do not practice safe sex.

Some populations are more at risk than others because they have an increased exposure potential. For example, coal miners are at greater risk for "black lung" disease than others because they are exposed to it more than others. Health care workers also have a greater exposure risk than other populations because of the nature of their occupation (sharps, HIV positive patients, etc.).

Relative risk ratios are statistical methods used in cohort and case series studies to determine risk cohort or case-series studies. Populations at risk, referred to as target groups, are targeted for intervention since they are at risk.

RISK STRATIFICATION

Risk stratification techniques profile individuals, groups and populations using several techniques such as threshold modeling, a clinical review and statistic modeling. Threshold modeling is done by including certain people, groups or populations who meet what is called inclusion criteria. When the individual or group is identified using these inclusion criteria they are then assigned to a particular healthcare intervention.

Clinical review involves selecting certain individuals, groups or populations and then having them further explored and examined using a clinical review to reconfirm their inclusion specifics, and eligibility to get a particular healthcare intervention. Statistical modeling uses the analysis of individual, group or population historical data to predict future occurrences and events for this individual, group or population.

Risks and the degree of risk are also attached to surgical procedures. The factors that impact on surgical infections include the site of the surgery and the degree of contamination that is innate to it, the length or duration of the surgery, and patient-related factors. For example, abdominal surgery, a surgical procedure that is longer than two hours in duration, a surgical site that is either dirty or contaminated before the surgery, and patients with three or more medical diagnoses are at greatest risk for surgical infections.

QUALITY

STRUCTURES, PROCESSES AND OUTCOMES

Measuring quality has evolved over the years, from quality control to quality assurance, then from quality improvement to performance improvement, and finally continuous quality improvement. It has also evolved from structure studies to process studies to outcome-related studies.

Successful quality management and performance improvement activities improve the outcomes of care, improve the safety and efficiency of processes, reduce costs and also reduce risks and liability.

These activities are mandated by external regulatory bodies such as the JCAHO, the Centers for Medicare and Medicaid (CMS) and state departments of health.

Although models differ somewhat, continuous quality or performance improvement activities include the identification of an opportunity to improve a process, organizing a team to work on the improvement activity (those closely related to the process must be included in the group), identifying customer expectations and outcomes, gathering data and information, including best practices and research studies, analyzing the data, close examination of the existing process, designing the process with measurable specifications that can be evaluated, the elimination of all variances, the implementation of the newly designed process, the evaluation of improvement in terms of the measurable specifications, and documentation of the entire procedure that led to the process change.

Efforts should focus on areas with the greatest risk, the greatest volume, the highest costs and the most problem prone.

QUALITY INDICATORS: CORE AND OUTCOME MEASURES

Quality indicators can be categorized as core measures and outcome measures.

Core measures are standardized measures of quality. JCAHO uses what are called ORYX National Hospital Quality Measures, which include measures of diseases like heart failure and pneumonia, population measures such as pediatric care, and organizational measures like those used in emergency departments.

Outcomes measures are used to examine the outcomes of care. For example, mortality and morbidity rates, infection rates related to hospital-acquired infections, lengths of stay and readmissions may be analyzed as outcome measures.

OUTCOME EVALUATION AND OUTCOME EVALUATION TOOLS

Structure, processes and outcomes can be evaluated with data.

Unfortunately, many infection control professionals want to measure outcomes without taking the necessary prior steps. When this is the case, outcomes will be unpredictable and filled with variances if the process and the structure are not stable. Unstable structures and processes will lead to unstable outcomes. The goal is to achieve and maintain stable and predictable high quality outcomes, so good structures and processes must be in place before outcomes can be optimized and stabilized.

Infection control professionals can and should measure outcomes relating to biological problems, psychological status, quality of life, functional abilities, the prevention of infections, goal attainment, safety, and the occurrence of adverse events.

Patient care practices, as well as the performance of the organization, can be measured and evaluated. This can involve the measurement of performance over time in a longitudinal manner to determine if planned changes have sustained increased performance, and measurements to identify problems and opportunities, then taking actions to strategically improve performance.

RISK MANAGEMENT

Risk management is closely aligned with continuous quality improvement, but instead of proactively planning change like quality improvement, risk management aims to reduce liability by eliminating risks and liabilities that can include patient related risks, quality risks and financial risks and liabilities.

Risk management identifies and eliminates hazards relating to basic safety such as falls, hospital-acquired infections and infant abduction, and a wide variety of medical errors such as wrong site surgery, wrong patient surgery and medication errors. JCAHO has requirements relating to medical errors in terms of reporting sentinel events and the elimination of hazards using root cause analysis.

The main concepts behind risk management include the identification of any potential risks that can occur, analyzing the likelihood of a risk occurring, what effects the risk can have, the cost associated with the risk, and consideration of how the risk can be controlled and, if possible, eliminated. Prevention of any and all negative outcomes that could potentially lead to a lawsuit or claim is necessary.

Infection control professionals must be able to identify patients who are vulnerable to high risk events, like infections. All patients should be screened for infection risk, and immediate and specific preventive measures should be put in place for all "at risk" patients.

ROOT CAUSE ANALYSIS

Root cause analysis is a process used to dig down to the deepest, real reasons why mistakes and errors have occurred. These reasons are usually procedures and processes and *not* people. Root cause analysis occurs in a blame-free environment with teams of stakeholders who closely analyze faulty processes with a number of techniques, such as brainstorming, flow charting, fishbone diagrams, data collection and statistical data analysis.

SENTINEL EVENTS

It is recommended that all sentinel events are examined using root cause analysis. A sentinel event is an occurrence that leads to, or has the potential to lead to, an adverse outcome. Even "near misses" are considered sentinel events. The processes that cause harm as well as those that lead to "near misses" must be refined and improved so that all possible human errors are eliminated and future sentinel events can be prevented.

Some of the most commonly occurring medical error sentinel events include the unintended retention of a foreign body after surgery or another invasive procedure, wrong patient/wrong site/ wrong procedure, treatment delays, suicide, operative and post-operative complications like infections, falls and other unanticipated events.

BENCHMARKING AND BEST PRACTICES

Benchmarking and the identification of best practices are superior ways that quality and risk can be objectively determined. Some hospitals provide less costly care, some achieve better patient outcomes and some have lower incidences of sentinel events. Infection control professionals should identify these best practices and attempt to replicate them in order to continuously improve quality.

VARIANCE TRACKING

In the context of continuous quality improvement, a variance is a quality defect. There are four types of variance:

- Practitioner variance
- System/institutional variance
- Community variance
- Patient/family variance

Variances can be random or specific. A random variance is one that occurs because of factors inherent to the process; these variances occur each time the established process is carried out. Specific variances occur due to one faulty part of the process. Both indicate that efforts must be made to correct and eliminate variance.

DATA MANAGEMENT

Data can be collected and analyzed to measure outcomes in terms of an individual or a group, population or aggregate. For example, an infection control professional can collect and use data to measure a program's effectiveness for a population, or the outcomes of care for a specific patient. The infection control professional may also use data to measure the clinical outcomes of care for a population, such as those affected with a postoperative infection.

IMPLEMENTING CHANGE

Once your research findings are clear, you will want to put your new knowledge to work improving patients' health care experiences. However, changing a system can be quite difficult – so difficult, in fact, that there is an entire academic field devoted to its study.

THEORIES OF CHANGE

In order for change to occur, the force of the facilitators to change must be greater in strength than the barriers to change; that is, the benefits must outweigh the costs. Change theories help us to understand and facilitate change, including corrective action plans, in our organizations.

LEWIN'S FORCED FIELD THEORY OF CHANGE

Lewin's Forced Field Theory of Change is perhaps the most popular of all change theories. Lewin's change theory consists of three phases of change: Unfreezing, freezing and refreezing. Lewin also describes barriers and facilitators to change.

1. *The Unfreezing Stage of Change.* During the unfreezing stage of change, there is awareness that there is a problem, need, or an opportunity that has to be addressed with some action. For example, the infection control professional may observe that the current outcomes of care do not currently meet expectations, established benchmarks and/or evidence based practices. The infection control professional is aware that there is a problem, and that there is a need, or opportunity, for improvement.

   This unfreezing process is challenging because many people and groups resist change and prefer the status quo. Resistance, nonetheless, can be overcome with things like motivational techniques, individual/group involvement and participation, and good communication. Humans are most apt to accept change when they understand and know that real benefits can result from the change.

2. *The Freezing Stage of Change.* During this stage, the planned change is implemented. Those affected by the change may experience feelings such as fear, uncertainty and resistance. These barriers, too, can be overcome with effective strategies like communication, education, and ongoing reinforcement of the fact that benefits will be realized.

3. *The Refreezing Stage of Change.* During the refreezing stage, the affected people have fully accepted and implemented the change. It becomes somewhat routine for them. Some of the factors that can positively affect this stage, in order to promote long lasting and sustained change, include support, continued positive reinforcement and stabilization of the change. The infection control professional also plays a highly critical role in the refreezing stage of change.

HAVELOCK'S SIX PHASES OF PLANNED CHANGE

The six phases of Havelock's Six Phases of Planned Change are developing relationships, diagnosing the existing problem, collecting available resources, choosing a solution, garnering acceptance and stabilizing the change.

LIPPITT, WATSON AND WESTLEY'S SEVEN PHASES OF CHANGE

Lippitt, Watson and Westley's Seven Phases of Change are patient awareness of the need for change, the development of a change agent/patient relationship, which includes the educator-patient relationship, the problem is defined, the goals are established, the plan for change is implemented, the change is accepted, and the change agent/patient relationship changes.

ROGER'S INNOVATION-DECISION PROCESS

The infection control professional, as change agent, provides others with knowledge and information about the benefits of change during the five stages of Roger's Innovation-Decision Process, which are knowledge, persuasion, decision, implementation and confirmation.

CHAOS THEORY

This change theory addresses the constantly changing environment and the way it affects the patient as an open system. Infection control professionals have to always expect the unexpected and never assume that predicted outcomes will occur automatically.

DECISION MAKING

Decisions, particularly complex and difficult ones, require much thought and collaboration in order to be sound and effective. At times, it is very difficult for teams to make a decision. If this is the case, more data collection and research may be indicated so that the pros and cons can be fully explored.

There are five unique different decision making processes that teams or groups use. The roles of the team leader and members differ in each of these:

- *Decide-* With this decision making process, the leader collects data and information from team members, but it is the leader, rather than the members, that make the final decision. After the decision is made, the leader simply informs the members about the decision.

- *An Individual Consultation-* The leader talks to each group member alone and never consults with the group as a whole during a group meeting. The leader then makes the final decision in light of the information obtained in this manner.

- *Group Consultation-* The group and the leader meet and to share information and opinions about the problem and possible solutions. After this group consultation, the leader comes to a decision.

- *Facilitation-* The leader takes on a cooperative holistic approach, collaborating with the group as a whole as they work toward a unified and consensual decision. The leader is non-directive and never imposes a particular solution on the group. In this case, the final decision is one made by the group, not by the leader.

- *Delegation-* The leader takes a backseat approach, passing the problem over to the group. The leader is supportive, but allows the group to come to a decision without their direct collaboration.

COMMON DECISION MAKING PROCESS

Although there are several decision making processes, the most traditional includes these steps:

1. *Identifying the purpose of the decision making*
    - What decisions are needed?
    - What has to be determined?

2. *Establishing criteria*
    - What is the desired outcome?
    - What must be avoided?

3. *Ranking and weighing criteria*
    - Which criteria are the most important?

4. *Exploring the alternatives in terms of the established criteria*
    - What are the alternatives in this situation?
    - Which alternatives have the greatest potential for success?

- Which alternative(s) is/are consistent with the established criteria?

5. *Exploring and forecasting potential risks and problems that could result from the selected alternative, or the course of action*

    - What are the risks?
    - What can be done to prevent or minimize the risk(s)?

6. *Implementation of the selected course of action*

    - The team observes the effects of the intervention

7. *Evaluating the outcome*

    - Have the pre-established goals been met?
    - Have these goals been met completely, partially or not at all?

THE PROBLEM SOLVING PROCESS

The problem solving process, similar to the decision making process, has these steps:

- *Problem Definition-* The most commonly occurring cause of problem solving failures is a failure to clearly define the problem. It is very important to separate the problem from the symptoms of the problem during this stage.

- *Data Collection-* Data and information relating to the problem at hand are collected and organized.

- *Data Analysis-* Data is analyzed during this stage and the initial problem definition is further refined as based on this data analysis.

- *Generating Possible Solutions to the Problem-* Open mindedness, creativity and the lack of bias can ensure a wide array of potential solutions.

- *Selecting the Best Possible Solution-* All potential solutions are considered after which the best possible solution is selected based on the benefit/risk ratio, its feasibility, its cost effectiveness, and other issues, such as legal and ethical concerns.

- *Implementing the Solution or Planned Change-* Leaders and others must evaluate the effects of this planned change as it is being implemented, rather than only waiting or doing nothing. Some solutions may lead to unanticipated risks and harm that must be immediately identified and corrected to ensure success.

- *Evaluating the Result of the Implemented Solution-* Has the change achieved the desired goal? Completely? Partially? Not at all?

EVIDENCE BASED PRACTICE

Evidence based practice is research based practice. Simply stated, evidence based practice begins with research, which is applied to the development and dissemination of evidence based practice guidelines through publications and professional conferences. These guidelines can and should be applied to practice after the research and the guidelines are critiqued by the infection control professional. Some areas of consideration for integrating evidence-based practices into one's role include:

- *Is the evidence based practice feasible and practical?*

- *Do the potential benefits of the evidence-based practice outweigh the possible risks and costs associated with its implementation?*

- *Is it potentially effective and efficient or is it too time consuming and limited in terms of effectiveness?*

Providing an evidence-based approach to care requires that you:

- *Access and appraise evidence (research findings)*

- *Understand the relationships between research and the strength of evidence*

- *Determine its applicability in respect to a particular patient's condition, context and wishes.*

RESEARCH DATABASES

- The Cochrane Library [6]

- The Agency for Healthcare Research and Quality National Guideline Clearing House [7]

- The Joanna Briggs Institute [8]

- Ovid's Evidence Based Medicine Reviews (EBMR) [9]

- Medlars [10]

- Medline Plus (An International nursing index and Index Medicus is also included) [11]

- Pub Med [12]

- The Cumulative Index to Nursing and Allied Health Literature (CINAHL) [13]

- The Directory of Open Access Journals (Free) [14]

---

[6] http://www.thecochranelibrary.com/view/0/AboutTheCochraneLibrary.html

[7] http://www.guideline.gov/

[8] http://www.joannabriggs.edu.au/

[9] http://www.ovid.com/webapp/wcs/stores/servlet/ProductDisplay?storeId=13051&catalogId=13151&langId=-1&partNumber=Prod-904410

[10] http://www.nlm.nih.gov/bsd/mmshome.html

[11] http://www.nlm.nih.gov/medlineplus/

[12] http://www.ncbi.nlm.nih.gov/pubmed/

[13] http://www.ebscohost.com/cinahl/)

[14] http://www.doaj.org

OUTBREAKS AND BREACHES

VERIFYING THE EXISTENCE OF AN OUTBREAK

An outbreak is defined as an increase in cases of disease in time or place that is greater than expected. The goals of outbreak investigation and management include:

- Decreasing the number of outbreaks by improving outbreak responses and preventive measures

- Identifying areas that need improvement in terms of outbreak prevention, outbreak identification and outbreak management

- To facilitate the collection, organization and aggregation of data in a standardized and centralized manner so this data is useful to others in terms of their infection control efforts

Outbreaks can be rare and unexpected; and they can have serious public health impacts. For example, a single case of measles as an act of bioterrorism can have serious impact. An outbreak is verified and confirmed when a laboratory test result confirms its presence.

Outbreaks are investigated and explored in terms of the etiology, their mode of transmission and the environment within which it exists. Is the etiology of the outbreak bacteria, viral, chemical or parasitic? What is the mode of transmission? Is it spread as a waterborne, foodborne, environmental of direct person to person contact pathogen? Is the outbreak occurring in a particular school, prison, long term care facility, hospital or restaurant?

Most unexpected outbreaks are foodborne, water borne, and vector borne; they are also primarily influenza type and respiratory outbreaks. Some may also occur when a vaccine preventable disease breaks out and others can be healthcare related.

Outbreaks are reported in terms of:

- The specific setting and location of the outbreak

- The number of people ill with the pathogen and the number of people who are susceptible
- The date that the outbreak was reported to local and state health
- The specific infectious disease etiology

The Centers for Disease Control and Prevention (CDC) and the National Outbreak Reporting System (NORS) recommends that outbreaks be reported with the following details:

- The name of the reporting agency and the date of the report
- Outbreak demographics including the number of cases, the gender and ages who those affected, the symptoms, the severity, the incubation period and the duration of the illness
- The name of the specific causal agent, chemical or toxin
- The exposure and transmission of the agent, the type of outbreak, setting, mode of transmission and the location or source of the outbreak
- The methods and techniques that were used to identify, explore, and investigate the outbreak

CASE DEFINITIONS AND FINDINGS

THE CASE DEFINITION

A case definition is a collection of uniform criteria that is used to define a disease, like an infectious disease, that can be subjected to surveillance. Case definitions are updated on at least an annual basis. Reportable diseases vary among the states of our nation; the Council of State and Territorial Epidemiologists (CSTE) recommends that state health departments report cases of diseases to CDC's National Modifiable Diseases Surveillance System (NNDSS).

Case definitions are classified and categorized by the CDC as below.

- *Confirmed case:* A case is confirmed for reporting

- *Epidemiologically linked case:* A case where a person who has had contact with a person, or persons, who has had the infection or was exposed to it and the transmission mode is plausible. An epidemiologically linked case can be linked to a laboratory confirmed case when the laboratory confirms at least one case in the chain of transmission

- *Clinically compatible case:* A clinical syndrome generally compatible with the disease, as described in the clinical description

- *Laboratory confirmed case:* A case which is confirmed with at least one laboratory method listed in the definition of the specific case as found under the Laboratory Criteria for Diagnosis despite the fact that other non-listed methods can be used for a clinical diagnosis

- *Probable case:* A case that is considered probable for reporting purposes

- *Supportive or presumptive laboratory results:* These laboratory results are used for, and consistent with, the particular diagnosis but they are not included in the specific laboratory results for the specified disease as found under the Laboratory Criteria for Diagnosis.

- *Suspected case:* A case that is considered suspected for reporting purposes

THE PERIOD OF INVESTIGATION

Epidemiologic studies and investigations of outbreaks can vary in terms of the duration of the study according the design and the purpose of the particular study. Outbreak investigations are conducted until the outbreak infection is identified and the source of the outbreak successfully reversed. At times, this can be a brief period of time and, at other times, this process can be quite lengthy.

CASE FINDING AND SCREENING

The purpose of case finding and screening is to identify a disease or infection among those in apparent good health who have an unrecognized disease or infection prior to the screening and case finding. These people, or populations, do not yet have any signs or symptoms associated with the disease or infection that is being screened for.

Screening attempts to identify possible disease in a community, population, or group early so that early prevention, intervention and management can reduce the risk of the disease or infection in terms of its morbidity and mortality. It should be understood, however, that not all screening techniques and tools are without intrinsic problems and concerns. Some screening may yield false negatives or false positive results that complicate the accuracy of the screening process. Over-diagnosis, under-diagnosis, misdiagnosis and a false sense of certainty may occur. Additionally, some screening processes can even have indirect and direct adverse effects on the individual, group or population being screened.

The ideal screening tool, therefore, should be inexpensive, safe, highly accurate, without adverse effects, highly sensitive to the disease or infection, and highly specific in terms of what it is identifying. Less than ideal screening can lead to unnecessary medical costs when a false positive screening occurs and people are treated; some adverse effects can include infection with invasive screening, anxiety from a false positive test, discomfort, pain and exposures to radiation and/or chemicals; and a false sense of security, as well as delayed diagnosis and treatment can occur with a false negative screening test.

There are several types of screening including universal screening, mass screening, high risk or selective screening and multiphasic screenings. Universal screening is defined as the screening of all individuals who are in a particular category according to established criteria. For example, all females may be screened, all children between 5 and 7 years of age may be screened, or all those in a hospital or long term care facility may be screened. Mass screening involves screening an entire group or population. High risk or selective screening is screening that is limited only to a population with a high risk; and, lastly, multiphasic screening is the use of more than one or multiple screening methods for the same disease or infection.

DEFINING THE PROBLEM: TIME, PLACE, PERSON AND RISK FACTORS

All investigations should be specific and narrow in focus, rather than vague and broad. For example, the problem that will be investigated should be clearly state in terms of time, place, person and risk factors.

The time of the investigation should be stated in terms of duration, the beginning date and time and the ending date and time. It should also be specific in terms of where the investigation will occur and in terms of the individuals, groups or population that will be investigated and those who are not included or delimited. For example, the group under investigation may include females with urinary tract infections between the ages of 70 to 74 except those who have an immunosuppressive disease. Those with immunosuppressive disease will be delimited and not included in the study.

Lastly, the known risk factors should be acknowledged and documented in the definition of the infectious disease problem that will be investigated and explored.

Hypotheses

A research or investigation question asks if there is a relationship among variables. A research question is composed with an interrogatory statement; a hypothesis is stated as a declarative statement.

Some examples of research questions are:

- "How does proper hand washing affect infection rates?"
- "What factors are impacting on the source of the infection?"

- "What is the mode of transmission for this specific pathogen in the community?"

- "What are the risk factors associated with hospital acquired respiratory infections?"

- "How does a systematic and complete surveillance program impact on the infection rates in the community?"

A hypothesis is defined as an "educated" prediction about the relationship between or among the variables under study. For example, an infection control researcher may state that "the rates of MRSA will rise according to the duration of a surgical procedure." Other possible hypotheses can state:

- The rate of surgical related infections will decrease with complete preoperative teaching

- The morbidity rate related to staph infections will decrease when the hospital uses established surveillance plans

- The severity of urinary tract infections will decrease with the limited duration of indwelling urinary catheters

- The mode of transmission will be eliminated with the decontamination of the community's water supply

- The pathogen source will be eliminated with the quarantine

No investigation or research study proves that the hypothesis is true or false. Research will only support or refute a hypothesis. For example, when the investigation finds that the mode of transmission was eliminated with the decontamination of the community's water supply, the hypothesis is supported; and when the source is not eliminated with quarantine, the hypothesis is not supported.

CONTROL MEASURES

Immediately upon the identification of an outbreak and its investigation, preventive and curative measures must be implemented. As these measures are implemented, ongoing evaluation to determine the effectiveness of the interventions are monitored in a continuous manner to ensure sustained success.

REPORTS

At the conclusion of the investigation, a final report must be prepared and disseminated, as indicated. For example, some reports are mandatory according to the state and other reports may be voluntary disseminated to a committee, a community group or the affected population(s). Sharing of knowledge and research is a professional responsibility.

INFECTION CONTROL BREACHES

Using the guidance of the CDC, infection control providers identify and implement actions when there has been an infection control breach. The steps of this process include:

1. *The Identification of the Infection Control Breach-* The type of biological matter or pathogen is identified, the nature of the breach is explored and the type of procedure that led to the breach is investigated. Additionally, the possibly infectious pathogens, bodily surfaces and areas, and possibly infected individuals and groups are identified.

   Whenever possible, immediate intervention and corrective actions are taken to reduce the risks associated with infection control breach. For example, the disinfection and sterilization processes may have to be corrected and those who came in contact with the contaminated device or piece of equipment should be identified.

2. *The Collection of Additional Data and Information-* After the particular infection control breach has been identified, it is

necessary to determine who has been affected. The infection control professional determines how many patients have been exposed, who these patients are, the time frame during which the breach persisted prior to its identification and correction, and the patients who have a history of infectious diseases such as HIV and/or hepatitis.

Medical history should be validated with public health surveillance records; when patient history is not clear or uncertain, the infection control professional may retrospectively review the patient's medical record to determine if the patient has a history of elevated liver transaminase, for example, which is a possible indicator of previously undiagnosed hepatitis B and/or hepatitis C.

In a large number of cases, the infection control professional should interview staff and personally observe the procedure led to the breach.

3. *The Notification of Stakeholders*- The next phase of the process includes the notification of stakeholders about the infection control breach. Examples of stakeholders include regulatory agencies, state and local departments of health, risk management personnel, all possibly affected healthcare workers and other infection control professionals.

4. *The Qualitative Determination of Risk*- Infection control breaches are then classified as Category A or Category B. Category A breaches are defined as breaches that result from gross error and/or a high risk practice that has a high possibility of exposure affecting others; Category B breaches are defined as less severe than Category A breaches where there is a lower possibility of exposure.

Some examples of Category A errors and breaches include any reuse of syringes and/or needles and/or the use of contaminated used needles for multiple dose vials and intravenous fluid bags. Because the aforementioned actions are grossly negligent, all healthcare providers who performed these actions should be reported to their licensing agency and terminated and/or disciplined according to the healthcare agency's policies and procedures.

Examples of Category B errors and breaches include incorrect endoscopic equipment disinfection and sterilization, including processing this equipment with the incorrect solution and/or with a briefer period of time than necessary.

5. *Patient and Patient Notification-* Decisions about who to notify are made. All Category A exposures should be followed up with patient or patient notification. Category B infection control breaches should be followed up with notifications as based on public health concerns and the potential for the risk of transmission to others.

Infection control programs should clearly address and delineate logistical issues, including communication and notifications, should an infection control breach occur. These infection control policies and procedures should address outbreaks, communication patterns and materials, guidelines for testing, post exposure prophylaxis, screening and counseling.

REPORTING AND NOTIFICATION

Breaches must be reported to the state's departments of health, and patients must be notified when there has been some compromise of a healthcare facility's infection control practices and procedures.

QUARANTINE

When the threat of contagious disease is present, the Centers for Disease Control and Prevention (CDC) as well as state and local laws, mandate that isolation and quarantine are initiated when indicated. Quarantine can be related to people as well as other things like buildings, animals and cargo when it is determined that these inanimate object have been contaminated with a contagious pathogen.

The primary difference between isolation and quarantine is that isolation applies to people who are ill with a contagious disease and quarantine applies to people and things that have been exposed to a contagious disease whether or not they are actually ill from it.

Quarantine is limited to those situations where a person, or a defined population, has been exposed to a highly contagious and deadly infection and there are available resources to adequately care for the patients and also maintain the quarantine.

Quarantine can become highly complex and complicated when, for example, a large number of people have been exposed to a highly contagious and serious infection while on an airplane or in a large public space like a sports stadium.

PREVENTING AND CONTROLLING TRANSMISSION

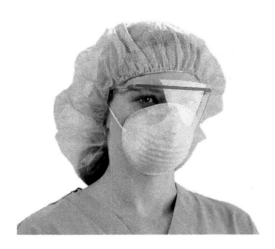

In this section, you will learn about how to develop and review complete and current infection prevention and control policies and procedures, how to collaborate with public health agencies in planning community responses to a wide variety of biological agents and how to identify and implement infection prevention and control strategies in this section.

CDC GUIDELINES

All healthcare facilities should follow CDC guidelines[15] for developing and reviewing infection prevention and control policies and procedures, found at:

These include:

- Preventing Healthcare-Associated Infections

- Guideline for Disinfection, and Sterilization in Healthcare Facilities

- Guidelines for Environmental Infection Control in Healthcare Facilities

- Guidelines for Hand Hygiene in Healthcare Settings

- Guideline for Isolation Precautions: Preventing Transmission of Infectious Agents in Healthcare Settings

---

[15] http://www.cdc.gov/hai/prevent/prevent_pubs.html#hhs

- Guidance on Public Reporting of Healthcare-Associated Infections: Recommendations

- Interim Guidance for Managing Patients With Suspected Viral Hemorrhagic Fever in U.S. Hospitals

- Guideline for the Prevention of Surgical Site Infection

- Guideline for Preventing Healthcare Associated Pneumonia

- Guidelines for Developing an Institutional Program to Enhance Antimicrobial Stewardship

- Management of Multidrug-Resistant Organisms in Healthcare Settings

- Guidance for Control of Infections With Carbapenem Resistant or Carbapenemase-Producing Enterobacteriae in Acute Care Facilities

- USPHS/IDSA Guidelines for the Prevention of Opportunistic Infections in Persons Infected with Human Immunodeficiency Virus

- Guidelines for Preventing the Transmission of HIV Through Transplantation of Human Tissue and Organs

- CDC's Perspectives in Disease Prevention and Health Promotion Update: Universal Precautions for Prevention of Transmission of Human Immunodeficiency Virus, Hepatitis B Virus, and Other Blood-borne Pathogens in Health-Care Settings

- CDC Recommendations for Prevention of HIV Transmission in Healthcare Settings

- USPHS/IDSA Guidelines for the Prevention of Opportunistic Infections in Persons Infected with Human Immunodeficiency Virus

The CDC device-associated infection prevention guidelines include:

- Guideline for Prevention of Catheter-Associated Urinary Tract Infections
- Guidelines for the Prevention of Intravascular Catheter-Related Infections

The CDC guidelines relating to employee health and occupational diseases include:

- Influenza Vaccination of Healthcare Personnel
- Guideline for Infection Control in Hospital Personnel
- Recommendations for Using Smallpox Vaccine in a Pre-Event Vaccination Program
- Updated US Public Health Service Guidelines for the Management of Occupational Exposures to Human Immunodeficiency Virus and Recommendations for Post-exposure Prophylaxis Infection Control and Hospital Epidemiology
- Exposure to Blood What Healthcare Personnel Need to Know
- Updated U.S. Public Health Service Guidelines for the Management of Occupational Exposures to HBV, HCV, and HIV and Recommendations for Post-exposure Prophylaxis
- Preventing Needlestick Injuries in Healthcare Settings
- Guidelines for Infection Control in Healthcare Personnel
- Evaluation of Safety Devices for Preventing Percutaneous Injuries Among Healthcare Workers During Phlebotomy Procedures
- Evaluation of Blunt Suture Needles in Preventing Percutaneous Injuries Among Healthcare Workers During Gynecologic Surgical Procedures

PREVENTION AND CONTROL STRATEGIES

HAND-WASHING

All healthcare workers must be educated about the need to wash their hands in the following circumstances:

- Before, during, and after preparing food
- Before eating food
- Before and after caring for someone who is sick
- Before and after treating a cut or wound
- After using the toilet
- After changing diapers or cleaning up a child who has used the toilet
- After blowing your nose, coughing, or sneezing
- After touching an animal, animal feed, or animal waste
- After handling pet food or pet treats
- After touching garbage
- As soon as one arrives at work
- Before entering a patient's room
- Before leaving the patients room
- Before you put gloves on and also as soon as you take the gloves off
- Before and after you touch anyone
- Before and after you perform any task
- Before and after you take a break
- Before you leave the restroom
- After handling trash
- After blowing your nose, coughing or sneezing
- Before and after eating or handling food
- When you are leaving work

They should also be taught about proper hand washing procedures:

- Wetting the hands with clean, running water (warm or cold), turn off the tap, and apply soap.
- Lather all hand surfaces thoroughly by rubbing them together and also under the nails.
- Vigorously scrub the hands for at least 20 seconds.
- Thoroughly rinse the hands well under clean, running water.
- Dry the hands using a clean towel, a paper towel or let them air dry.

Proper hand-washing procedure is important and it should only take about 20 seconds. Try singing the "Happy Birthday" song twice – that's about 20 seconds.

HAND SANITIZERS

Although hand sanitizers can rid the hands of a large number of microbes, they do not eliminate all types of pathogens. Hand-sanitizers should not be a substitute for good hand-washing; the only time they should be used is when hand-washing facilities are not accessible.

CLEANING, DISINFECTION AND STERILIZATION

TERMINOLOGY

In addition to the basic terminology listed on page 13, you must become familiar with the following terms:

- *Autoclave*: a device that sterilizes instruments or other objects using steam under pressure. The length of time required for sterilization depends on temperature, vacuum, and pressure.
- *Bactericide*: an agent that kills bacteria.

- *Biofilm*: the accumulated mass of bacteria and extracellular material that is tightly adhered to a surface and cannot be easily removed.

- *Contact time*: the time a disinfectant is in direct contact with the surface or item to be disinfected. For surface disinfection, this period is framed by the application to the surface until complete drying has occurred.

- *Control, positive*: a biologic indicator, from the same lot as a test biologic indicator that is left unexposed to the sterilization cycle and then incubated to verify the viability of the test biologic indicator.

- *Detergent*: a cleaning agent that makes no antimicrobial claims on the label. They are comprised of a hydrophilic component and a lipophilic component, and can be divided into four types: anionic, cationic, amphoteric, and non-ionic detergents.

- *D value*: the time or radiation dose required to deactivate 90% of a population of the test microorganism under stated exposure conditions.

- Endoscope: an instrument that allows the examination and treatment of the interior of the body canals and hollow organs.

- *Flash sterilization*: the process designed for the steam sterilization of unwrapped patient-care items for immediate use (or placed in a specially designed, covered, rigid container to allow for rapid penetration of steam).

- *Fungicide*: An agent that destroys fungi (including yeasts) and/or fungal spores pathogenic to humans or other animals in the inanimate environment.

- *General disinfectant*: An EPA-registered disinfectant labeled for use against both gram-negative and gram-positive bacteria. Efficacy is demonstrated against both Salmonella and Staphylococcus. Also called broad-spectrum disinfectant.

- *Germicidal detergent*: A detergent that is also an EPA-registered disinfectant.

- *High-level disinfectant:* An agent capable of killing bacterial spores when used in sufficient concentration under suitable conditions. It therefore is expected to kill all other microorganisms.

- *Inorganic and organic load:* naturally occurring or artificially placed inorganic (e.g., metal salts) or organic (e.g., proteins) contaminants on a medical device before exposure to a microbicidal process.

- *Intermediate-level disinfectant:* An agent that destroys all vegetative bacteria, including tubercle bacilli, lipid and some non-lipid viruses, and fungi, but not bacterial spores.

- *Limited disinfectant:* A disinfectant registered for use against a specific major group of organisms (gram-negative or gram-positive bacteria). Efficacy has been demonstrated in laboratory tests against either Salmonella or Staphylococcus.

- *Lipid virus:* A virus surrounded by an envelope of lipoprotein, in addition to the usual core of nucleic acid, surrounded by a coat of protein. This type of virus (e.g., HIV) is generally easy to inactivate with many types of disinfectants. Also called enveloped or lipophilic virus.

- *Low-level disinfectant:* An agent that destroys most vegetative bacteria, some fungi and some viruses, but not resistant microorganisms like spores or mycobacteria.

- *Minimum Effective Concentration (MEC):* The minimum concentration of a liquid chemical germicide needed to achieve the claimed microbicidal activity, as determined by dose-response testing. Sometimes used interchangeably with Minimum Recommended Concentration.

- *Non-lipid viruses:* Generally more resistant to inactivation than lipid viruses. Also called non-enveloped or hydrophilic viruses. They can be inactivated with a one-step disinfection process: the simultaneous cleaning and disinfection of a noncritical surface or item.

- *Parametric release*: The declaration that a product is sterile on the basis of physical and/or chemical process data, rather than on sample testing or biologic indicator results.

- *Sanitizer*: An agent that reduces the number of bacterial contaminants to safe levels, as judged by public health requirements. Commonly used with substances applied to inanimate objects. According to the protocol for the official sanitizer test, a sanitizer is a chemical that kills 99.999% of the specific test bacteria in 30 seconds under the conditions of the test.

- *Spore*: A relatively water-poor round or elliptical resting cell consisting of condensed cytoplasm and a nucleus, surrounded by an impervious cell wall or coat. Spores are relatively resistant to disinfectant and sterilant activity and drying conditions (specifically in the genera Bacillus and Clostridium).

- *Steam quality*: A steam characteristic reflecting the dryness fraction (weight of dry steam in a mixture of dry saturated steam and entrained water) and the level of non-condensable gas (air or other gas that will not condense under the conditions of temperature and pressure used during the sterilization process). The dryness fraction (i.e., the proportion of completely dry steam in the steam being considered) should not fall below 97%.

- *Steam sterilization*: A sterilization process that uses saturated steam, under pressure for a specified exposure time and at a specified temperature, as the sterilizing agent.

- Steam sterilization, dynamic air removal type: One of two types of sterilization cycles in which air is removed from the chamber, and the load is inactivated by a series of pressure and vacuum excursions, or by a series of steam flushes and pressure pulses above atmospheric pressure (steam-flush-pressure-pulse cycle).

CLEANING

Simply stated, cleaning is the eradication of extraneous material from objects, including the supplies and equipment used in healthcare. Cleaning agents typically include water and a detergent, or soap, or with the use of water and a cleaning enzyme.

Thorough cleaning is necessary before disinfection and sterilization and it is also necessary when a single-use piece of equipment, such as a bedpan or urinal, is used. The purpose of cleaning all material prior to disinfection and sterilization is to remove all organic and inorganic materials so they do not interfere with the sterilization process. For example, surgical instruments are soaked, cleaned and rinsed prior to the sterilization process.

Cleaning can be done manually or with a mechanical device like an ultrasonic cleaning unit. Manual cleaning uses the friction, scrubbing rubbing and rinsing. When a mechanic device is used for cleaning, the instruments should be disassembled whenever possible, and items should not be stacked. These actions facilitate adequate contact with the cleaning agent.

DISINFECTION

Disinfection is the chemical or thermal destruction of pathogens and other microorganisms. Disinfection is more rigorous than cleaning, but it is less effective and deadly than sterilization, which unlike disinfection, kills all bacterial spores. The "ideal" disinfectant is:

- Rapid acting
- Environmentally safe
- Odor free
- Inexpensive
- Broad in terms of its antimicrobial actions
- Immune to factors such as the presence of organic material
- Nontoxic to patients and healthcare professionals
- Not harmful to any surfaces such as metals and plastics
- Thorough and not able to leave any residual film

- Highly soluble and stable in a dilutant

Disinfectants can be classified according to their form, such as liquid or a gas, or according to their spectrum of activity, such as a high level, intermediate level or low level of broad-scoped actions. They can also be classified according to their mechanisms of action, as well as their actions on cell membranes and cellular proteins.

Disinfectants must be tested in terms of their efficacy using one or more of the following tests:

- Rideal Walker Method
- Chick Martin test
- Koch's method
- Capacity use dilution test (Kelsey-Sykes test)
- In-use test

STERILIZATION

Sterilization processes can be chemical, physical, or a combination of both. Effective sterilization requires consistent and continuous operator competence, proper cleaning, wrapping, loading the sterilizer, and ongoing evaluation of the entire process.

Equipment is completely inspected and tested using tests like the Bowie-Dick test, as well as biological and chemical indicators that should all be negative.

Central supply and processing departments typically have separate areas for decontamination, sterilization, packaging and storage that are separated by physical barriers. For example, the decontamination area may have negative pressure, so that any contaminated airflow cannot enter other areas. All areas are highly restricted in terms of who enters.

Physical items entering the area are considered contaminated; therefore, protective personal equipment like gloves, gowns, tongs for sharps, face masks, and eye protection such as goggles or full-length face shields are used when handling these items.

After items are cleaned, dried, and thoroughly inspected, they are wrapped in preparation for sterilization. Hinged items are opened, removable parts are taken apart, items with concave surfaces are placed carefully to enable drainage, and items are not stacked in the sterilizer. Packaging ensures that sterility can be achieved with the penetration of the sterilant. Sequential and non-sequential double wrapping is often performed.

The sterilizer is loaded to permit the proper circulation of the sterilization agent. Sterile items can be stored for varying amounts of time. For example, they will remain sterile for as long as 9 months when a 3 mil heat sealed pack is used, and they will remain sterile for 30 days when wrapped in double thickness muslin. Sterile items can be stored with the date of sterilization and its expiration date or when an event related shelf live which deems things as sterile until an event, like a package tear or moisture.

Sterile supplies are stored at least 10 inches from the floor, 2 inches from the wall and 18 inches from the ceiling (which should have sprinkler heads) so that the supplies have adequate ventilation.

The entire sterilization process is closely monitored with mechanical, chemical, and biological indicators. Mechanical monitoring entails the daily assessments of temperatures, pressures and cycle time; reactive ink chemical indicators are placed inside the pack to ensure sterility; and biological indicators, the most rigorous of monitoring tools, provide sterility information as soon as the sterilization process is done.

These indicators test for the presence of hardy, difficult to kill spores, enzymes and/or metabolites. A negative biological indicator indicates that the item is sterile. A single positive spore test does not necessarily indicate a sterilizer failure, but the sterilizer must be immediately re-challenged; if it is still positive, the sterilizer must be taken out of service and all items in it are considered contaminated.

Some examples of sterilizing agents and processes include:

- *Peracetic acid* is an oxidizing agent that removes surface contaminants like protein found on endoscopic tubing. This agent oxidizes sulfhydryl and sulfur bonds in proteins, enzymes, and other metabolites, and it stops cell wall permeability.

- *Ionizing radiation* is a low temperature sterilization technique that employs electron accelerators or cobalt 60 gamma rays. It is rarely used because it is very expensive and, according to the CDC, there are no FDA-cleared ionizing radiation sterilization processes for use in healthcare facilities. Radiation sterilization is often referred to as "cold sterilization" because it does not employ the use of heat.

- *Dry heat sterilization* is used only when the equipment or supply can become damaged and unusable when it is subjected to moist heat. For example, sharp instruments can become dull with moist heat. The two types of dry heat sterilizers are the forced air type and the static air type.

- *Liquid chemicals* are used for sterilization; however, when compared to thermal sterilization, they do not penetrate as well. Chemicals are typically restricted for the sterilization of items that are heat-sensitive and not able to be sterilized in another manner.

- *Vaporized hydrogen peroxide* equipment uses relatively rapid vacuum systems, accommodates most materials and is relatively simple to use and operate. Some studies have found vaporized hydrogen peroxide to be effective against MRSA, serratia marcescens, clostridium botulinum spores and clostridium difficile.

- *Ozone* is an effective oxidant created by the sterilizing machine with self-contained biological and chemical indicators. After the process is completed, the ozone converts back to water vapor and oxygen. This type of sterilization technique can be used for a wide variety of materials and it is effective even with very resistant microorganisms.

- *Gaseous chlorine dioxide* is a rapid form of sterilization typically taking only about 30 minutes. It has no mutagen or carcinogenic effects on humans.

- *Heat* is perhaps the most reliable method of sterilization, provided that the item can be subjected to it. Heat coagulates proteins and has an oxidative effect. Dry heat is less effective than moist heat; and the time of sterilization has a negative correlation with the amount of time needed to sterilize. For example, as the temperature increases, the time necessary for sterilization decreases. The time and temperature necessary for sterilization has to be increased as the number of microorganisms increase and the resilience of the organisms increases. For example, spores are the most resilient and resistant.

- *Autoclave sterilization* is commonly used in healthcare. An autoclave uses the combination of heat and pressure. Many items can be rendered sterile in as little as 15 minutes using an autoclave and the steam is much more penetrative than dry air.

INFECTION CONTROL IN GENERAL PATIENT CARE AREAS

Infection control is particularly challenging when direct and indirect patient care areas are not controlled. General patient care units are subjected to heavy traffic and individuals from the external environment. Some of these individuals and visitors may have communicable diseases and can serve as a mode of transport of pathogens. For example, a visitor may enter the patient care area with clostridium difficile on their hands; as they enter the unit, they have contact with doors, door knobs, rest rooms, the cafeteria and other areas of the hospital. Although many healthcare agencies place masks and hand sanitizers at the entry to the unit, many people ignore their use and enter without using these patient protection items.

INFECTION CONTROL IN THE OPERATING ROOM

The operating suite is a particularly high-risk area in terms of infection control. The CDC has infection control guidelines related to the operating suite environment and its practices. For example, the CDC states that the amount of microbial skin, respiratory and dust will increase, according to the number of people moving about in the area. Operating rooms should use positive air pressure (to decrease air from moving from "dirty" or less clean areas to more clean areas) as well as HEPA filters, ultraviolet radiation and laminar airflow systems to control and eliminate pathogens in this sterile areas.

Operating room surfaces such as floors, lights and walls should be routinely cleaned after each surgical procedure; tacky mats are placed at entries, and routine microbiological sampling and testing are done to monitor the surgical environment. Surgical attire should be addressed in the facility's policies and procedures relating to the proper laundering of this attire.

The Association of Operating Room Nurses and OSHA recommend that scrub suits are immediately changed if they appear soiled. Other personal protective equipment includes masks, surgical caps or hoods, shoe covers, sterile gloves which are best doubled, gowns, drapes and, of course, surgical asepsis.

Some of the evidence-based practices relating to traffic in the preoperative area include paperless electronic documentation, an intercom or video communication system, and surgeon and procedure-specific preference cards to ensure the availability of necessary supplies and equipment. All of these measures, and others, decrease the need for frequent door openings and closings, as well as unnecessary traffic in the highly infection prone operating suite.

Asepsis, specifically surgical asepsis, is the cornerstone of safe, infection-free surgical and invasive procedures. Maintaining homeostasis while preserving adequate blood supply, removing devitalized or necrotic tissues, using drains and suture material appropriately, preventing hypothermia, gently handling tissues, eradicating dead space, and appropriately managing the postoperative incision are all necessary to prevent infection.

It appears that monofilament sutures have the lowest infection rates when compared to other kinds of sutures. At times, drains are separate from the incision site to prevent infection; closed, rather than open, drains are preferable. Additionally, drains should be left in place for the briefest period of time as possible. The presence of hypothermia from general anesthesia also appears to increase the risk of a surgical incision infection. .

INFECTION CONTROL AND THERAPEUTIC PROCEDURES

DIALYSIS

Patients who undergo dialysis treatment have an increased risk for getting a healthcare-associated infection (HAI). Hemodialysis patients are at a high risk for infection because the process of hemodialysis requires frequent use of catheters or the insertion of needles to access the bloodstream. Also, hemodialysis patients have weakened immune systems, which increase their risk for infection, and they require frequent hospitalizations and surgery, where they might acquire an infection.

The CDC recommends vaccinations for patients with pre-end-stage renal disease including the hepatitis B vaccination in higher dosage than normal, with serologic follow up to determine if revaccination is necessary and perhaps even an annual booster dosage. Additionally, hemodialysis patients are routinely tested for the presence of hepatitis C.

ENDOSCOPY

Although the complications of endoscopy have a low rate of incidence, an infection introduced by the endoscope and a piercing or tear of the area being examined may occur.

Generally speaking, endoscopic infections are typically associated with failures to follow establish disinfection and sterilization policies and procedures. The most commonly occurring infections typically include blood-borne pathogens such as hepatitis B and C, particularly with a gastrointestinal endoscopy.

The single most important thing that can be done to prevent these infections is the scrupulous and proper reprocessing and disinfection of endoscopes.

The American Society for Gastrointestinal Endoscopy recommends:

- *Mechanical Cleaning*

  The internal and external portions of the endoscope must be thoroughly washed with a detergent containing enzymes and thorough brushing.

- *Disinfection*

  After thorough mechanical cleaning is done, the endoscope is soaked with an FDA approved disinfection chemical for a period of time.

- *Post Processing Treatment*

  After disinfection, the endoscope is rinsed thoroughly with water to remove any debris and residual chemicals, after which it gets a final alcohol rinse and thorough drying using forced air.

BRONCHOSCOPY

Although the rate is low with bronchoscopy, infection is most often secondary to a preexisting infection in the upper respiratory tract that pushes downward during the procedure, contaminating instruments, solutions and other equipment used during the procedure. This type of contamination, although rare, does occur, perhaps due to a loose fitting or another area that could not be properly disinfected and sterilized.

Some of the infections associated with bronchoscopy include Pseudomonas aeruginosa, Serratia marcescens, non-tuberculosis mycobacteria and environmental fungi.

URINARY DRAINAGE CATHETERS

Urinary catheterization for residual urine may be used, as well as an indwelling urinary catheter. However, whenever possible, catheterization should be avoided in order to prevent urinary tract infections. Catheter-associated urinary tract infections (CAUTI) are a major concern in healthcare. All invasive procedures and treatments, such as inserting catheters, place the patient at risk for infection. These infections can affect any area of the urinary system, including the bladder, ureters, urethra, and kidney. The prevention of catheter-associated urinary tract infections includes:

- Inserting and using urinary catheters only when necessary
- The removal of the catheter as soon as possible
- The insertion, care and maintenance of the catheter by competent staff
- Maintaining unobstructed urinary flow
- Maintaining a closed urinary drainage system without disconnecting the catheter from tubing or the tubing from the drainage bag
- Securing the catheter to the leg to prevent pulling on the catheter
- Avoiding any kinking or twisting of the catheter
- Always keeping the catheter and bag lower than the level of the bladder to prevent any urinary backflow
- Keeping the bag lower than the bladder to prevent urine from back flowing to the bladder
- Emptying the collection bag frequently and not touching the drainage spout with anything.

Some alternatives include a portable ultrasound device to assess urine volume, and antimicrobial-impregnated catheters, such as silver-alloy coated catheters, to reduce the risk for catheter-associated urinary tract infections by eliminating the need for catheterization and to prevent infection, respectively. Additionally, external condom catheters should be considered for male patients and intermittent catheterization, rather than an indwelling catheter, should also be considered.

INTRAVASCULAR DEVICES

Intravenous catheterization with a central line, including with peripherally inserted central catheters (PICCs), is more risky than peripheral intravenous lines; however, these too can lead to infection.

Thrombosis and bloodstream infections are two of the most serious of all vascular access complications, and infections are the most serious of all. Vascular access device infections have a high morbidity and mortality rate. They are also costly in terms of human suffering. The "ideal" intravenous catheter should be:

- Inexpensive
- Resistant to thrombosis and infection
- One with a long dwell time without the danger of infection
- Antimicrobial and impregnated with broad scope antiseptics like chlorhexidine in its materials and along its entire length

RECALLS

Recalls are mechanisms that remove products, foods, and medical equipment from use when they are contaminated or unsafe. Despite the voluntary nature of most recalls, the vast majority of manufactures and producers remove contaminated and/or dangerous items from use in order to ethically preserve health and safety as well as to avoid litigation. When they fail to voluntarily recall a product, the FDA can issue a recall order according to their Medical Device Recall Authority, so long as a risk to health exists. The FDA's recall classifications are Class I, Class II and Class III:

- *Class I Recalls* - This classification involves products that have a reasonable probability that their use will cause serious adverse health consequences or death.

- *Class II Recalls* - Class II recalls involve those products that that may cause temporary or reversible adverse health consequences or where the probability of serious adverse health consequences is not probable and remote.

- *Class III Recalls* - These products are not likely to cause adverse health consequences.

When a company recalls a product or piece of equipment, it must inform the consumer, or healthcare organization, about the recall product in terms of its size, lot, serial numbers and other identifying information. They also have to advise the consumer about the reason for the recall, inform them that further use or distribution should immediately stop, and give instructions about how the product should be disposed of, returned or repaired with corrective action.

ISOLATION AND BARRIER PRECAUTIONS

Most healthcare infections are spread by the hands of health care workers from one patient to another. These infections are limited to only those that a patient did not have before they were hospitalized, or cared for, but were acquired after admission or after care was provided.

The most commonly occurring risk factors for these infections are prolonged illness and immunosuppression, which can result from an infection like HIV, treatments such as chemotherapy, and some medications. All equipment and non-sterile supplies can harbor and spread pathogenic infections.

The urinary tract, the respiratory tract, wounds, and the bloodstream are the most common sites for healthcare acquired infections; some of the commonly occurring pathogens include E. coli, Candida albicans, staphylococcus aureus, pseudomonas aeruginosa, and enterococcus.

Hand washing is the single most effective way to prevent nosocomial infections. Protective standard and transmission-based precautions are also necessary to prevent the spread of infections, which is doubly important due to the presence of so many resistant strains of pathogens, like MRSA, VRE and penicillin-resistant strep.

Protective precautions include:

- *Standard precautions* that apply to all blood and bodily fluids and all patients regardless of the person's diagnosis.

- *Contact precautions* to prevent any direct and indirect contact transmissions, as those contained in diarrhea, wounds, and herpes simplex.

- *Airborne precautions* for the prevention of airborne transmission microbes like TB. These include a HEPA mask and a negative pressure room.

- *Droplet precautions* to prevent the transmission of pathogens through a cough or sneeze. Masks are indicated for these precautions.

PLACEMENT

Patient placement is integral to the healthcare facility's infection control policies and procedures, particularly when an outbreak of an infectious disease occurs or a patient, or group of patients, has an infectious, contagious infection.

Cohorting patients is one method. Cohorting patients entails the purposeful clustering and grouping of patients in one room or area when one or more patients are infected with the same infectious agent, to prevent the spread of infection to others, particularly those who are susceptive to infection. Cohorting staff is the assignment of staff to care for cohorting patients with the same infectious disease in order to prevent the spread to other patients who are not infected and can be susceptible to the infection.

ENVIRONMENTAL HAZARDS

Airborne pathogens like Mycobacterium tuberculosis and varicella-zoster virus, and environmental pathogens like Aspergillus and Legionella, can lead to serious illnesses among healthcare workers and patients alike unless they are prevented with engineering controls and environmental infection control strategies.

Preventive measures include the appropriate use of disinfections and other cleaners, the proper cleaning and maintenance of equipment, particularly endoscopic and hydrotherapy equipment, maintaining high quality water standards, particularly in hemodialysis settings where water quality determinations are necessary, maintaining ventilation standards, particularly when airborne infection can occur and preventing any water intrusion into the healthcare setting.

The CDC recommends:

- Ongoing monitoring of water and ventilation systems

- Multidisciplinary teams to perform ongoing infection control risk assessments

- Physical barriers and dust control measures during all repairs and construction of the physical environment

- Special preventive environmental measures for physical areas that have patients who are at high risk for infection

- Air filtration systems and airborne-particle sampling to monitor the effectiveness of air filtration and dust-control measures

- Established procedures to ensure the health and safety of patients in the operating rooms when a patient with infectious tuberculosis needs surgery

- Routine culturing of water as part of a comprehensive control program for legionellae when indicated

- Established procedures relating to water supply problems including water leaks, flooding and disruptions of the water supply

- Special management and preventive measures for water supply to problem prone areas and pieces of equipment like ice machines, hemodialysis machines, hydrotherapy equipment, dental unit water lines, and automated endoscope preprocessors

- Disinfection and surface cleaning of environmental surfaces that are effective against all antibiotic resistant pathogenic microorganisms

- Infection control procedures and preventive measures for the management of health-care laundry

- Established infection control policies and procedures that address animals that are used for therapy and as a service animal

Healthcare facilities should also monitor and determine the effectiveness of their environmental health program, policies and procedures. Questions to ask include:

- Are infection control staff involved in the risk assessment and daily monitoring of the presence of negative pressure in construction and renovation areas?

- Is the facility performing monthly assays to monitor for endotoxins in water for reprocessing of hemodialyzers?

- Is the facility performing monthly assays to monitor for mesophilic and heterotrophic bacteria in the water used for the preparation of dialysate and for the reprocessing of hemodialyzers?

- Is the infection control program effective in terms of determining and correcting possible environmental sources of non-tuberculosis mycobacteria with cultures of water and laboratory specimens?

IMMUNIZATION PROGRAMS

The CDC requires healthcare facilities to protect personal health and to protect the health of other patients and residents with immunization surveillance and the provision of protective immunizations, as indicated.

This surveillance requires that all facilities determine whether or not patients meet the criteria for the seasonal annual vaccination during the influenza season, from September to April of each year. They also recommend that healthcare facilities provide other vaccinations, such as the Hepatitis B, MMR, Varicella and Pneumococcal vaccinations; these requirements vary from state to state with exemptions for medical, religious and philosophical reasons.

Some exemptions include an allergy to the components of the vaccination, a previous history of Guillain-Barre syndrome within 6 weeks after an immunization and/or a current temperature of 101.5 degrees. Some personal exemptions include a fear of injections, a profound fear of side effects and a perceived belief that immunizations are ineffective. Some of the religious exemptions include religious beliefs and practices that prohibit the use of vaccines.

INFECTION CONTROL AND EMERGENCIES

All healthcare facilities have internal and external emergency preparedness plans. Internal disasters include events like fire, the loss of electricity, the loss of communication systems and a bomb threat or actual bomb explosion. External disaster plans cover events in the community that bring large numbers of victims into the healthcare facility. Some external disasters include events like major train or plane accidents and the massive use of bioterrorism agents in the community. For more information on bioterrorism, see the next chapter.

BIOTERRORISM

Bioterrorism is defined as the intentional, malicious and planned release of an infectious agent into the community to cause panic, fear, terror and illness among people, vegetation and/or animals. These bioterrorism agents include a wide variety of pathogens including bacteria, viruses and chemical toxins that can be transmitted in a number of ways including with the food and water supply, in the air and with human contact.

The CDC, the American Red Cross, the American Medical Association, The US Food and Drug Administration, the National Library of Medicine/National Institutes of Health, and the US Environmental Protection Agency, among other associations and organizations, provide a wide variety of guidance for infection control professionals, laboratory professionals, healthcare providers and those who work with the water and food supply.

All healthcare facilities are required to have emergency preparedness plans to address acts of bioterrorism such as:

- Anthrax
- Arenaviruses
- Botulism
- Brucellosis
- Chlamydia psittaci
- Cholera
- Epsilon toxin
- Q fever
- Ebola virus hemorrhagic fever
- Nipah virus and hantavirus
- Tularemia
- Lassa fever
- Marburg virus hemorrhagic fever
- Melioidosis
- Plague
- Psittacosis
- Ricin toxin
- Shigella
- Smallpox
- Staphylococcal enterotoxin B

- Typhoid fever
- Typhus fever
- Viral encephalitis

CLASSIFICATIONS OF BIOTERRORISM AGENTS

The CDC classifies bioterrorism agents in three categories: A, B and C.

CATEGORY A BIOTERRORISM AGENTS

Category A bioterrorism agents are the most lethal of all categories. They pose the greatest possible threat in the community because they are associated with a high mortality and morbidity rate; they are easily and quickly spread to others with human contact; and they can lead to short term and long term public health destruction.

Tularemia

Tularemia, also known as rabbit fever, is associated with a high degree of dysfunction but a low morbidity rate. Tularemia is transmitted to humans with inhalation, ingestion, and insect bites. Without prompt diagnosis and treatment, people who inhale this infectious agent experience life threatening respiratory compromise and sepsis.

Anthrax

Unlike many other infectious bioterrorism pathogens, anthrax is only transmissible through direct contact with the spore-laden bacteria. Early treatment includes an antibiotic such as ciprofloxacin.

Smallpox

This virus is highly contagious and rapidly transmitted in the air from person to person; smallpox is associated with a high mortality rate when left untreated. Globally, it can be prevented with a vaccine but the immunity is limited, so revaccination is often indicated, particularly since this infection is reemerging as a public health threat.

Botulism

The clostridium botulinum is one of the most lethal of all toxins. It can lead to paralysis and respiratory system collapse and death.

Viral Hemorrhagic Fever

Viral hemorrhagic fevers are caused by a number of pathogens in the Filoviridae and Arenaviridae family, which includes the Ebola virus. Ebola has a mortality rate of up to 90% and, at the current time, there are no cures or treatments other than supportive care. The cause of death among those affected with this virus is multisystem failure and/or hypovolemic shock.

Bubonic Plague

The bubonic plague, also known as the "Black Death" or "Black Plague," was responsible for the deaths of *hundreds of millions* people in Europe, Asia and the Islamic world. In the 15th century, it killed over 60% of Europe's population. Many people erroneously believe the disease is extinct, but the truth is that the Black Plague is still alive and well – and the last epidemic of it actually struck America, afflicting hundreds of people. Anywhere between five and fifteen Americans contract bubonic plague every year, usually by rodents, flea bites and in contaminated aerosols.

CATEGORY B BIOTERRORISM AGENTS

These are the second most lethal bioterrorism agents – they spread quickly and cause moderately high morbidity and mortality rates. Like Category A bioterrorism agents, they pose a public health threat, but the degree is lesser. Examples include:

Salmonella

The vast majority of salmonella infections occur as the result of ingesting contaminated foods. The two types of salmonella include non-typhoidal, which is the most commonly occurring type and typhoidal salmonella. Non-typhoidal salmonella is typically self-limiting and it can be spread between animals and human beings.

Typhoidal salmonella occurs only in humans and leads to typhoid fever, which negatively affects multiple bodily organs, including the kidney and liver. Sepsis occurs when the endotoxins affect the nervous and vascular systems, leading to both septic and hypovolemic shock.

Shigella

Shigella is transmitted via the fecal–oral route, ingestion. It affects humans and other primates. Shigella can lead to severe diarrhea and dysentery and, as such, is most threatening to infants, children and the elderly. It can be treated with medications such as ciprofloxacin and ampicillin, as well as intravenous fluid replacement, when diagnosed early in the course of this infectious disease. Antidiarrheal medications are not indicated because these pharmacological interventions can worsen the disease.

Brucellosis

Brucellosis, also referred to as undulant fever, rock fever, Malta fever, Bang's disease and Crimean fever, is ingested by humans in dairy products and contaminated meats as well as transmitted with human to human contact.

Some of the signs and symptoms of brucellosis include joint pain, muscular pain and weakness and severe diaphoresis; some of the complications of brucellosis are uveitis, endocarditis, leucopenia, thrombocytopenia, spondylitis, severe neurological complications, meningitis and granulomatous hepatitis.

A combination of antibiotics such as rifampicin, streptomycin and tetracycline are effective when administered after prompt diagnosis. This infection can also relapse after a period of time, so close monitoring is essential. When death occurs, it is most commonly the result of endocarditis and cardiovascular compromise.

Q Fever

Q fever, caused by the Coxiella burnetii bacterium, can affect domestic and wild animals as well as humans. Q fever is transmitted via inhalation and, in some cases, the bite of an infected tick.

The signs and symptoms include fever, muscular pain, anorexia, severe diaphoresis, upper respiratory and sometimes severe gastrointestinal respiratory problems, although some patients may be asymptomatic. Some life threatening complications include acute respiratory distress syndrome (ARDS), granulomatous hepatitis, hepatomegaly, endocarditis and atypical pneumonia.

The treatment of Q fever includes antimicrobial medications such as tetracycline, ciprofloxacin, ofloxacin, chloramphenicol and hydroxychloroquine.

Psittacosis

Psittacosis, also referred to as ornithosis and parrot fever, is caused by the Chlamydophila psittaci bacteria and, in nature, it is transmitted by birds.

This signs and symptoms of this potential bioterrorism agent include some that mimic meningitis and typhoid fever. They include a high fever, diarrhea, arthralgia, leucopenia, Horder's spots (rosy-colored skin spots,) splenomegaly, nuchal rigidity, pneumonia, and coma in severe cases. Some of the complications associated with this infectious disease include encephalitis, myocarditis, endocarditis, and hepatitis.

The treatment of choice is chloramphenicol and tetracycline intravenously or orally. When tetracycline is contraindicated, as it is among pregnant women and children less than nine years of age, erythromycin is used.

Ricin

Ricin is a highly lethal, carbohydrate-binding protein that can be deadly when ingested or particularly so when inhaled. Without successful treatment, ricin can lead to severe diarrhea, shock and death.

The signs and symptoms vary according to the form. Inhaled ricin can lead to dyspnea, chest tightness, fever, hypotension, pulmonary edema and respiratory failure. Ingested ricin can lead to nausea, vomiting, bloody diarrhea, dehydration, hypotension, seizures, multisystem failure and death. Cutaneous and eye exposure lead to skin or eye redness.

With cutaneous and eye exposure, ricin should be immediately washed off. Ingested ricin should be rid from the body as soon as possible with gastric lavage and activated charcoal; inhaled ricin often necessitates supportive life saving measures such respiratory assistance, intravenous fluids, seizure prevention and the management of the patient's blood pressure. There is no cure or antidote for ricin toxicity.

Staphylococcus Enterotoxin B

Staphylococcus enterotoxin B is an extremely hardy staphylococcus that affects the gastrointestinal tract with nausea, cramping, diarrhea, extensive inflammation, and can lead to antibiotic resistant strains, including those that lead to toxic shock syndrome.

Some of the signs and symptoms associated with staphylococcus enterotoxin B include a characteristic "sunburn" type rash, skin peeling or desquamation, hypotension, fever, confusion, stupor, multisystem failure, coma and death when left untreated. Treatment typically includes hospitalization and supportive care in terms of hydration, respiratory status, renal care and the prevention of life-threatening complications. The pharmacological treatment of staphylococcus enterotoxin B is a combination of antimicrobial agents such as penicillin, vancomycin, cephalosporin, clindamycin and gentamicin.

Typhus

In nature, typhus is transmitted by fleas, rats, and other animals like raccoons and skunks. Typhus, which is not the same as typhoid fever, is caused by the rickettsia bacteria.

The signs and symptoms of murine or endemic typhus are backache, abdominal pain, a diffuse red rash, coughing, nausea, muscular pain, joint pain, and a very high fever of up to 106 degrees. The signs of epidemic typhus include coughing, delirium, a fever of up to 104 degrees, joint pain, severe muscular pain, changes in mental status like confusion and stupor, hypotension, a diffuse rash and sensitivity to light.

Some of the complications of typhus include pneumonia, renal impairment and damage to the central nervous system. The treatment includes antimicrobial therapy with medications, such as tetracycline, doxycycline and chloramphenicol.

Viral Encephalitis

A wide variety of viruses including measles, herpes simplex, mumps, rabies, the West Nile virus and rubella can lead to encephalitis in addition to acts of bioterrorism, contaminated foods, inhalation, insect bites and skin contact.

The signs and symptoms of viral encephalitis include cerebral edema, brain damage, changes in levels of consciousness and cognition, a high fever, confusion, nuchal rigidity, sensitivity to light, stiffness, intracerebral hemorrhage, paralysis, stupor, seizures, permanent brain and death.

The goals of treatment include the maintenance of life and central nervous system functioning as well as the prevention of long term complications, such as paralysis and incapacitating brain damage. Supportive treatments include fluid replacement, nutrition and rest to conserve central nervous system functioning.

Antiviral pharmacological interventions including foscarnet and acyclovir, and anticonvulsants like phenytoin. Steroids like dexamethasone to reduce brain inflammation, as well as sedation, are often indicated.

CATEGORY C BIOTERRORISM AGENTS

Although a threat to public health, Category C bioterrorism agents are less lethal and threatening than Categories A and B agents. This category includes new and emerging threats that can be easily produced and released in the future. The CDC identifies the Hantavirus and the Nipah virus as examples of Category C bioterrorism agents. Other new and emerging diseases include SARS and influenza H1N1.

INFECTIOUS DISEASE CONTROL PROGRAMS

All healthcare facilities should also have infectious disease control programs that interrelate and interact with other agencies. Some of these threats include all infection outbreaks including those relating to influenza, meningitis and hepatitis. At times, the state departments of health and the Centers for Disease Control and Prevention are agencies that infection control professionals interact with.

OCCUPATIONAL HEALTH PROGRAMS

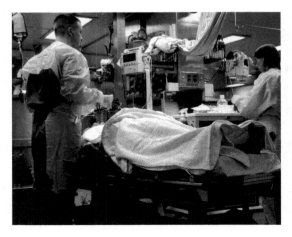

This section will teach you the essential components of a thorough, effective occupational health program. This includes information about screening and immunization, counseling, follow up, work restriction related to communicable diseases, analysis and trending of occupational exposure incidents, and how to assess related risks.

SCREENING AND IMMUNIZATION

The CDC has infection control guidelines that directly apply to hospital personnel. The purpose of these guidelines is to protect the healthcare staff from the transmission of infections and also to protect the consuming public from infections that can be transmitted to them by healthcare providers. Some of these guidelines include immunizations for preventable diseases, like influenza, isolation procedures and personal protective equipment to protect the healthcare provider, and the management of post exposure prophylactic interventions when a healthcare worker has been exposed to an infectious disease and also work restrictions when a worker is affected with a communicable disease. Required components include medical evaluations, immunization programs, coordination with other departments such as the laboratory and nursing departments, the provision of infection control and safety education, training and counseling for new and existing employees, maintaining medical records, and insuring the privacy and confidentiality of staff medical records.

Medical evaluations should be done prior to the hiring and placement of new personnel. A complete health history, including immunization status and preexisting medical conditions, is collected and a complete physical examination should be done.

Screening may be necessary to determine the prospective employees' level of immunity to vaccination-preventable diseases such as measles, mumps, hepatitis B, rubella, and/or varicella. Tuberculosis screening is routinely prior to employment and throughout the course of employment in a healthcare facility.

The immunizations for healthcare personnel must include the hepatitis B vaccine, the MMR vaccine and an annual influenza vaccination. Other vaccines that should be made available to some staff in special circumstances include the BCG vaccine for tuberculosis, hepatitis A, meningococcal polysaccharide, polio, rabies, tetanus and diphtheria, and smallpox vaccines, when indicated.

Some other major considerations that must be included in the employee health program include the mechanisms that are used for post exposure prophylaxis when a healthcare worker is exposed to a serious pathogen such as:

- Diphtheria
- Hepatitis A
- Hepatitis B
- Meningococcal disease
- Pertussis
- Rabies
- Varicella-zoster virus

STAFF TRAINING AND COUNSELING

TRAINING AND EDUCATION

Personnel will be more apt to comply with the infection control program when they are educated about it, and when there are established policies and procedures in place that ensure the efficiency and effectiveness of infection control practices and procedures.

Education and training should address the individual's roles, responsibilities and related infection control practices that will protect the worker and the patients that are cared for in the healthcare facility. Some employees will need more technical and advanced education than others; some may require that the infection control practitioner modify the teaching in order to meet specific learning needs in terms of language, terminology and level of complexity.

HEALTH COUNSELING

Health counseling is also an integral part of the employee health program. According to the CDC, health counseling should provide mechanisms with which healthcare staff can learn about occupational infections, the risks and prevention associated with healthcare related infections, the risks associated with occupational exposures, how the healthcare organization manages exposures, methods of post exposure prophylaxis, and how to prevent the transmission of pathogens within the family and in the community.

JOB-RELATED ILLNESS

Employee job related illnesses and exposures to occupational hazards have to be treated and managed. At times, decisions about possible work restrictions have to be made to protect the health and safety of the affected individual, the other staff and the patients. Work restriction should be based on a number of different factors, including the nature of the employee's job, the mode of transmission of the offending pathogen and the cause of the illness or exposure.

Policies and procedures concerning job-related illnesses and exposures should be carefully designed so that employees are encouraged to report these events without adverse consequences, such as the loss of salary and/or job status, while preserving the protection of others. This employee protection is particularly important because, among other things, employees are not legally able to collect workers' compensation benefits as a result of infectious disease. Established employee health programs should therefore provide a mechanism for the continuation of salary, benefits and job status when it is necessary to restrict work.

Work restrictions, when necessary, should apply to all staff including department heads. Some examples of infectious diseases that can, and should be, reported 24 hours a day and seven days a week include things like diarrhea, conjunctivitis, cytomegalovirus, herpes, all forms of hepatitis, diphtheria, and salmonella.

Policies and procedures should be specific in terms of the restriction. For example, some infectious diseases should exclude all patient contact, all contact with the patients' environment, contact with handling food, a restriction in terms of high risk patients, restrictions from contact with some populations like neonates and those with an immunosuppressive disorder.

The duration of the work restriction should also be addressed. For example, the work restriction can continue until the symptoms cease, until a culture is negative on a minimum of two specimens, or until a certain number of days after the onset of symptoms, like a rash, have occurred.

OCCUPATIONAL HEALTH ADMINISTRATION

RECORD KEEPING

As with all patient information and records, confidentiality must be ensured and continuously maintained. The CDC provides guidance in terms of these records, and OSHA mandates their confidentiality, employees' rights to access them, their retention for at least 30 years after employment has ceased, and complete, accurate and current record keeping.

Data should be maintained in a manner that provides readily available information about individuals and groups in terms of:

- Physical medical examinations and evaluations

- Immunization history and immunizations provided during the course of employment

- Any exposures that have occurred

- All post-exposure prophylaxis

STUDYING EXPOSURE INCIDENTS

The collection, analysis and trending of occupational exposure incidents should be a collaborative process with the infection control professional and various departments and individuals within the facility.

Some of these entities and individuals should include members of the occupational health department, the infection control department, the quality assurance and performance improvement department, the risk management department and affected individuals and groups, such as nurses, laboratory workers and physicians.

LEADERSHIP, MANAGEMENT AND COMMUNICATION

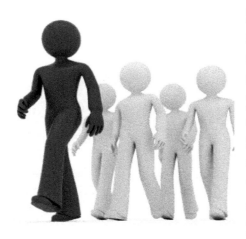

Professionals working in infection control must be managers, leaders and effective communicators in order to be successful. This section will give you the knowledge, skills and abilities to plan and develop an infection control program, communicate and provide feedback to others and develop, implement, and evaluate quality and performance improvement activities.

LEADERSHIP AND MANAGEMENT

Leadership is a complex concept that is difficult to fully define. Although definitions vary, leadership is a complex activity that involves empowering, inspiring, motivating, influencing, and guiding others to achieve goals.

Although many equate leadership with management, they are quite different. Management, simply defined, is organizing, planning, directing and controlling movement towards goals and objectives; and leadership is guiding and influencing others to accomplish goals.

Stephen R. Covey has defined and described the eight characteristics of successful and effective leaders as those who:

1. Are service-oriented

2. Are synergistic thinkers who view the whole as greater than the sum of its parts

3. Seek out and actively engage in lifelong learning
4. Believe in other people
5. Transmit positive energy that motivates others
6. Are committed to the common good
7. View life as a challenging adventure and they lead a balanced life
8. Actively engage in their own self renewal

Many agree that the underlying attribute of leaders is emotional intelligence. Emotional intelligence has five domains: Empathy, managing one's emotions, self-awareness, self-motivation and success in interpersonal relationships.

Other traits and attributes that leaders possess are integrity, a high level of energy, trustworthiness, optimism, courage, superior decision making and critical thinking skills, perseverance, the acceptance of accountability and responsibility, and superior communication, coaching and counseling skills. Some of the barriers to leadership include the lack of necessary personal, financial and administrative support resources. Many believe that people in power are leaders and also that people are born leaders, neither of which are true.

LEADERSHIP THEORIES

The three major theories of leadership can be classified as situational, attitudinal, and trait:

- *Situational theories of leadership* are based on the premise that leaders respond with certain behaviors according to the particular situation. Some examples of situational theories of leadership include Hersey and Blanchard's Situational Leadership Theory, the Contingency Theory and the Path Goal Theory.

- *Attitudinal theories of leadership* are based on the premise that leaders respond and act according to their attitudes rather than a situation. The Ohio State Leadership Studies Theory and the Michigan Leadership Studies Managerial Grid are examples of attitudinal theories of leadership.

- *Trait theories* support the idea that leaders, their attributes and traits define the leader and their actions, rather than other factors or forces that inspire others. Some examples of trait theories include the Charismatic Theory, the Great Man Theory and the Attribution Theory.

OTHER LEADERSHIP THEORIES

Transformational Leadership

Transformational theories, also known as relationship theories, focus upon the connections formed between leaders and followers. At the current time, Transformational Leadership is considered to be one of the best of all forms of leadership.

Transformational leaders motivate and inspire others with a shared vision; they have high expectations of others and themselves; and they are adept at setting clear goals and managing conflicts.

The four major components of this theory include idealized influence that allows others to act like the leader with their role modeling, individualized consideration of others as unique individuals, inspirational motivation that is possible with a shared vision and intellectual simulation which stimulates others to innovate and produce.

The Learning Organization Theory

The leader, according to this theory, is a visionary who aims to create a learning organization with a shared vision. These organizations continuously evolve and transform, because constant learning occurs among all members of the group or the organization. A Learning Organization has five components:

1. *Systems Thinking* - Organizations are open, interconnected systems. Changing a part changes the entire system and the environment.

2. *Personal Mastery* - All members of the organization are committed to learning.

3. *Mental Models* – Examples of mental models include collective memories and cultural norms that perpetuate certain values, behaviors, practices, and norms. Learning organizations challenge mental models, discard them and form new ones that are consistent with the learning organization.

4. *Shared Vision* - Shared vision offers organizations and groups a common identity and, in a learning organization, the shared vision is continuous learning. The strongest and most powerful of all visions is built on the individual visions of members at all levels of the organization; these visions are hampered when traditionally structured upper level management, or any other level, impose visions. Because of this, most learning organizations have decentralized, flattened tables of organization rather than traditional, hierarchical and unyielding, inflexible structures.

5. *Team Learning* - Team, or shared, learning is the sum of individual learning. Team learning occurs when members cross boundaries, such as departmental boundaries, in an atmosphere that facilitates and motivates members to open dialogue with others. This leads to improved problem solving skills and the dissemination of knowledge.

Advantages of learning organizations include increased efficiency, increased responsiveness to changes in the environment and within the organization, and improved quality outcomes. Barriers to creating a learning organization include the lack of an organizational commitment to learning, and the tendency of large, complex organizations to have difficulties with true, ongoing knowledge sharing.

Likert's Leadership Styles Theory

This theory is focused around the idea that, if leaders build affinity with their followers or subordinates, they will be more able to create and maintain a work environment that is effective, productive and capable of goal achievement. Likert described the types of leaders as:

1. *Exploitative-Authoritative*: Leaders motivate others with punishments, fear and threats. This type of leadership is the most controlling of the four types of leadership, according to Likert. This style often leads to worker hostility, anger and a lack of commitment to goals. In this style, the leader makes all of the decisions and they are usually not aware of problems that actually exist at the front line.

2. *Benevolent-Authoritative*: This style has less punishment and more rewards than the exploitive authoritative style of leadership. It also includes more participation of staff at the lowest level and more leader awareness of problems at the lower levels. Decisions are still made by the leader rather than made in a participative manner. Communication moves from the top to the bottom; little communication goes upwards. Staff often experience low satisfaction, hostility, and compromised productivity.

3. *Consultative*: This style facilitates higher levels of motivation, increased job satisfaction and greater productivity than the benevolent-authoritative and authoritative-exploitative styles of leadership. Punishments decrease, rewards increase, communication moves freely both downward and upward and the workers have more of a role in problem solving and decision making.

4. *Participative*: This style is the most effective and satisfying of all because there is full participation in decision making and a reward system is in place.

Lewin's Leadership Theory

According to Lewin, there are three primary leadership styles:

1. *Autocratic Leadership (Authoritarian)*: Autocratic leaders make independent decisions without communicating, collaborating and consulting with others. This style is indicated in emergency situations when there is no time for discussion and participation; however, when it is used for other situations, such as planned change, it causes the workers to be unmotivated, demoralized, uncreative and lacking of a sense of ownership.

2. *Democratic Leadership (Participative)*: Leaders provide guidance to members and get worker input in the decision making process. As a result, team members tend to have high levels of job satisfaction, creativity, motivation, engagement and productivity. Although it is a time consuming type of leadership, it is highly effective and beneficial, particularly when changes are indicated.

3. *Laissez-faire Leadership (Delegative)*: These leaders give team members a great amount of freedom and autonomy in terms of what, how and when tasks are done but they are readily available to provide necessary resources, including guidance and support when needed. This style facilitates high satisfaction, increased productivity and the abilities to perform independently and autonomously.

Goleman, Boyatzis and McKee Six Leadership Styles

1. *Visionary*: The leader articulates the goals but not the process to reach them. This leadership style leads to risk taking, creativity, and innovation.

2. *Coaching*: The leader's coaching maximizes the connection of the individual's personal and job-related goals to the person's unique strengths.

3. *Affiliative*: The leader demonstrates genuine empathy to create harmonious relationships within the group.

4. *Democratic*: The leader collaborates with members of the team, and they collectively and collaboratively resolve conflicts to achieve goals.

5. *Pacesetting*: The leader increases levels of performance and influences others to work more effectively and more efficiently.

6. *Commanding*: This style is the least effective. The commanding leader mandates compliance without explanations, and control and monitor groups very closely.

The Leadership Style Matrix

Flamholtz and Randle's theory states that leaders should select the best style to use after considerations relating to the group members, their level of competency and the nature of the situation and the task at hand.

1. *Work-Related:* This category is comprised of two tasks:

    - *Goal Emphasis*: The leader focuses on communicating and monitoring pre-established goals.

    - *Work Facilitation*: The leader obtains and provides the resources necessary to accomplish the goals.

2. Group Member Needs: This category is comprised of three tasks:

    - *Interaction Facilitation*: The leader facilitates relationships that are effective, respectful and mutually satisfying for all members. The leader monitors communication patterns and interactions.

    - *Supportive Behaviors*: The leader increases others' feelings of value, self-worth and importance.

    - *Personnel Development*: The leader provides ongoing support so the individuals can continue to grow and develop in order to reach their highest possible levels of potential.

COMMUNICATION

Communication is the act of conveying a message to another person with the use of writing, speech, behaviors, and pictures. Communication is a dynamic, interactive, and highly active process during which messages are formed by the sender, transmitted by the sender and received by the receiver of the message. Communication allows individuals to transmit, or convey, meaning, information, emotions, and beliefs. Humans initiate and maintain connectedness with others when they communicate.

THE COMPONENTS OF THE COMMUNICATION PROCESS

The components, or elements, of the communication process are the:

- Sender
- Receiver
- Message
- Channel
- Feedback or response
- Variables
- Encoding
- Decoding

The sender transmits the message to others; the receiver is the person who gets the message from the sender. The sender and receiver alternate roles throughout a conversation as they respond and provide feedback to each other. The channel is the means by which the message is conveyed or transmitted from the sender to the receiver. Examples of channels are using vision and using touch. The message is the feelings or information that is transmitted from the sender to the receiver.

A verbal or non-verbal response sent from the receiver to the sender after a message is called feedback. Feedback allows us to acknowledge the fact that the message was received, to respond to the message, to seek clarification of the message and/or to convey an understanding of the message. Feedback helps the sender of the message to validate that the message was accurately received and interpreted by the receiver of the message.

Encoding and decoding take place during communication Encoding is the cognitive process that the sender uses when contemplating how they will frame or formulate the message. Decoding is the cognitive process that the receiver uses in order to comprehend the message that is received from the sender.

Some of the factors that affect the communication process include language, values, distractions, perceptions, cultural background, and emotions.

LEVELS OF COMMUNICATION

There are six levels of communication:

1. *Intrapersonal Communication*: Intrapersonal communication is internal self-talk and thought. This level of communication helps the person to critically think, to resolve internal conflicts, to evaluate their own personal behavior and feelings, to self-reflect, and to meditate. Intrapersonal communication, unlike other forms of communication, does NOT transmit a message to another person or group.

2. *Interpersonal Communication*: This type of communication, which occurs between people, can occur face-to-face or through the use of the telephone or another electronic medium, such as a text message. Interpersonal communication is the main feature of the therapeutic patient relationship. It facilitates the transmission of many types of messages.

3. *Small Group Communication*: Small group communication is defined as communication that occurs among three or more people who have a common purpose or goal. This type of communication normally occurs face-to-face, but may also occur as a conference call or a video link. Infection control professionals often employ small group communication when they conduct a small group teaching session with a group of

patients who share a common illness and similar educational needs.

4. *Organizational Communication*: Organizational communication is used when a company or a hospital, for example, disseminate information to members of a specific organization.

5. *Public Communication*: Public communication is defined as communication that occurs with a large group of people. Healthcare professionals often participate in seminars and conferences, which are examples of public communication.

6. *Mass Communication*: Occurs when a small number of message senders communicate with a large and anonymous audience using media such as the television or the newspaper.

POSITIVE AND NEGATIVE FACTORS ON THE COMMUNICATION PROCESS

Some of the factors that can positively and negatively impact on the communication process include:

- Cultural values and beliefs
- Perception
- Attitudes
- Differences in knowledge
- Past experiences
- Emotions
- Relationships and roles
- Environmental settings
- Physical discomfort
- Time pressures

The infection control professional must establish and maintain therapeutic, open and nonjudgmental relationships with patients and staff members that are culturally sensitive and culturally competent. Cultural values or beliefs often differ between patients and healthcare professionals; different worldviews, vocabulary and terminology affect human interactions and communication.

Perceptions and attitudes also influence how a message is interpreted. Effective and therapeutic communication can also be quite challenging when the sender and receiver differ in terms of their levels of education and knowledge. Because the vast majority of patients, and significant others, do not understand medical terminology, anatomy, physiology and disease processes, healthcare professionals should avoid medical jargon and communicate with patients in a manner that is fully understandable to the patient and significant others.

Past experiences can also powerfully affect perceptions and interpretation of the meaning of messages. Patient's negative past experiences with healthcare systems can lead to skepticism and a lack of trust. Additionally, many emotions can influence how a person relates to others. Fear, pain, anger, and anxiety often adversely impact on the infection control professional-patient interaction and communication.

Relationships and roles directly affect the style and type of communication. For example, some cultures hold the male as the primary decision maker and some patients withhold personal details about themselves until trust and a nonjudgmental relationship is established.

The healthcare environment is not particularly conducive to good communication. Infection control professionals must attempt to control the environment where there is privacy, and make it comfortable and free of noise or distractions, in order to facilitate optimal communication with patients and significant others.

Physical discomfort, fatigue, pain and anxiety adversely impact on the communication process. Whenever possible, these factors should be minimized or eliminated to facilitate a good therapeutic relationship with the patient.

The pressure of time and urgency to complete other tasks while communicating with patients interferes with effective communication. For example, a patient will not fully discuss their needs, feelings, fears and concerns when they perceive that the infection control professional is in a hurry.

VERBAL AND NONVERBAL COMMUNICATION

VERBAL COMMUNICATION

People simultaneously employ both verbal and non-verbal types of communication. Verbal communication, which is typically conscious, transmits messages by speech.

Some of the components of verbal communication include sounds like crying and groaning, the tone, pitch and intonation of the sender's voice, the volume of speech, the rate or pace of the speech, the simplicity of the speech, the use of pauses, the clarity of the speech, the brevity of the discussion, the credibility of the message sender and the appropriate use of humor.

Sounds are often difficult to accurately interpret. Often, sounds can convey or express several emotions. Expressionless speech conveys a lack of interest to the patient; a loud voice and rapid speech is often highly intimidating. Pauses can help the sender and the receiver of the message to think about the message and encode feedback; prolonged pauses can be awkward and uncomfortable for the patient.

Short, clear and simple messages are more easily comprehended by the patient, and are less prone to misinterpretation and misunderstandings. The infection control professional - patient communication pattern must also be adaptable according to the patient's needs. For example, the infection control professional will alter their tone from cheerful to compassionate when the patient is expressing pain. Open, honest and nonjudgmental communication fosters the infection control professional's credibility and reliability. Lastly, humor is therapeutic when indicated; t can decrease stress and anxiety.

NONVERBAL COMMUNICATION

Nonverbal communication is far less conscious than verbal communication. Many consider nonverbal messages stronger and more powerful than the words that are transmitted concurrently with a verbal message. The factors that affect nonverbal communication are:

- Gestures
- Touch
- The use of space
- Bodily movements, or body language
- Facial expressions
- Eye movements
- Body posture and gait
- Personal appearance
- Congruency with the verbal message

Individuals communicate many feelings, emotions, and attitudes with their body movements, body language, and gestures. The way that a person holds themselves, walks, stands, sits, and moves about can communicate negative feelings and emotions such as depression, fatigue, a lack of interest, pain and despair; conversely, these factors can send a message of self-confidence, high self-concept, sense of wellbeing, and a positive and optimistic mood.

Eyes and eye movements are very revealing and reflective of a number of different things. Direct eye contact can convey openness, sincerity, a positive sense of self and interest. Conversely, a lack of eye contact can convey shyness, nervousness, embarrassment, dishonesty, defensiveness, and low self-esteem.

Touch or tactile communication conveys caring, compassion, and understanding. However, healthcare professionals must be aware that some individuals and cultures are not accepting of touch by members outside of their immediate family unit.

Facial expressions can transmit and convey happiness, sadness, surprise, impatience, disgust, fear, boredom, and anger, among a wide variety of other emotions. An emotionless face indicates a flat affect that may be the result of a lack of interest, some type of illness such as severe depression or Alzheimer's dementia, or it may be the patient's usual expression. Additionally, healthcare professionals must be constantly aware of their own facial expressions, other forms of nonverbal communication, and the effect they can have on patients and their family members.

Communicating with a patient at eye level, rather than an upper position, makes the patient more comfortable and able to openly communicate with the infection control professional or other health care workers. This conveys equality, nonjudgmental attitudes, and interest in the healthcare professional-patient relationship.

Personal appearance strongly influences the initial first impressions and perceptions that people form about others. Some of the things that provide this nonverbal data include manner of dress, style of hair, makeup and degrees of cleanliness.

On occasion, the spoken word and the nonverbal message sent with facial expressions or other forms of nonverbal communication do no match. They are incongruent. It is then, up to the healthcare professional, to decipher the meaning of both messages and clarify the meanings of both with the patient.

PERSONAL SPACES

All individuals have a personal bubble of space around them that dictates their level of comfort when others invade it. Although these personal spaces vary among individuals, situations and cultures, there are four general categories.

THE INTIMATE ZONE

This space ranges from 6 inches to 1½ feet from the body surface. This space is reserved for those who have an intimate relationship with the individual and infection control professionals who have to invade this personal space when performing many aspects of care, such as wound care or obtaining a laboratory specimen. We must approach the patient with a full explanation of what will be done and, at the same time, ensure the patient's comfort and bodily privacy when invading the intimate zone.

THE PERSONAL ZONE

This space extends beyond the intimate zone, defined as from 1½ feet to 4 feet from the person's body surface. The person zone is entered with social gatherings.

THE SOCIAL ZONE

This zone is typically permissible by individuals during interactions with strangers, and it ranges from 4 feet to 12 feet.

THE PUBLIC ZONE

The public zone, which is over 12 feet, is the distance that people normally choose when they are addressing, or speaking to, a large group of people.

THERAPEUTIC COMMUNICATION

Some therapeutic communication skills are described below:

SEEKING CLARIFICATION

Clarification is necessary in order to ensure that the patient and the healthcare professional fully understand each other's messages without making any premature or faulty assumptions. Clarifications can be done with direct and indirect statements and questions, such as "What did you mean about…" or "Tell me more about…."

PROVIDING LEADS

Infection control professionals should encourage patients to openly express their feelings and communicate their messages.

Providing leads like, "Tell me more about your fears" is a lead that is open-ended and conducive to patient communication.

PARAPHRASING

Restating and paraphrasing allows the healthcare professional to acknowledge an understanding about what the patient has said and meant in their sent message.

LISTENING

Active listening is far more than hearing; it is an active process that involves full engagement and a full interpretation of the nonverbal and verbal messages.

PRAISE AND ACKNOWLEDGMENT

Praise and acknowledgement are positive reinforcers that motivate a patient to continue moving towards their expected goals.

SILENCE

The use of therapeutic silence is particularly helpful when the patient is expressing deep and profound thoughts, feelings and beliefs that do not necessitate a response. Prolonged silence, however, may be uncomfortable or perceived as a lack of interest.

REFLECTION

This form of therapeutic communication mirrors the patient's feelings, not words, back to the patient so they can further explore these feelings with the healthcare professional. For example, when a patient expresses anger towards a son because he has not visited for days, the infection control professional may say, "You seem upset today. Would you like to talk about it?"

PERCEPTION VALIDATION

This is similar to clarification in terms of purpose. The infection control professional, for example, may ask the patient to talk about their feelings and beliefs so the infection control professional can validate what they perceive they have heard from the patient.

OFFERING OF SELF

Infection control professionals offer themselves unconditionally to the patient in a compassionate and caring manner.

FOCUSING

This form of therapeutic communication enables the patient to better focus on and present their main thoughts and ideas so it can be fully understood by the infection control professional.

Other components of a therapeutic infection control professional-patient relationship and communication are the establishment of trust, the fostering of open and honest communication, the encouraging of patient expressions of feelings, beliefs and views, the provision of an environment that is unconditionally accepting and respectful, and maintaining a nonjudgmental, unbiased attitude towards the views, feelings, situations and ideas of patient regardless of whether or not the infection control professional agrees with them.

BARRIERS TO THERAPEUTIC COMMUNICATION

Barriers to therapeutic communication and conversation stoppers include changing the subject, defensiveness, false reassurances, probing, disagreeing, judgments, rejection and challenging.

People change the subject inappropriately when they are unwilling or too uncomfortable to discuss the subject at hand. It stops the conversation. For example, a patient may perceive that the healthcare professional is not interested in or concerned about their feelings or beliefs when the healthcare professional changes the subject because of their own anxiety and discomfort.

"Don't worry, you will be just fine" is an example of false reassurance. Healthcare professionals often give false reassurances due to a personal inability to emotionally cope with the patient's state of health, fears and feelings. False reassurances can lead the patient to experience further anxiety and may cause the patient to feel as though the healthcare professional does not care about them.

Defensiveness enters interactions when the healthcare professional feels a need to defend themselves and/or the healthcare system for weaknesses and shortcomings.

Challenging occurs when the healthcare professional directly or indirectly asks the patient to justify and defend their beliefs, thoughts, and feelings. Challenging attacks the patient and the validity of the patient's own thoughts and feelings.

Probing is invasive and it violates the patient's right to privacy. Testing is also not therapeutic. Testing occurs when the healthcare professional asks a question that the patient is forced to answer with a response that is beneficial to the healthcare professional and not the patient. For example, the healthcare professional may state ask, "Do you think that I am taking good care of you today?" The patient is forced to say "yes".

Stereotyping is a barrier to effective communication because it entails general statements that do not reflect individuality. Both disagreement and insincere expressions of agreement also block open, therapeutic communication. All patient feelings and beliefs are valid - not right or wrong.

Lastly, judgmental attitudes force the patient to believe that they must agree with the healthcare professional and change their own personal beliefs and concerns.

ORGANIZATIONAL COMMUNICATION

Communication connects people in the organization together; it can transmit rules, responsibilities, regulations, and feedback; it is essential to information sharing and the coordination of functions.

Problems related to organizational communication are often deeply rooted and potentially lead to uncertainty, decreased decision making, problem solving and productivity. They also lead to poor planning and sometimes, even hostility. Effective communication and the climate within which it occurs should be clear, understandable, and congruent with the organization's actions, and should include attentive listening.

FORMAL AND INFORMAL PATTERNS

There are two basic types of organizational communication: Formal and informal patterns.

Formal communication patterns transmit organization-wide information relating to goals, procedures, policies and news along the linear (top to bottom) channels of communication established in the table of organization. Informal communication patterns can run in all directions. Informal lines, or chains, of communication are often referred to as the "grapevine"; at times, this "grapevine" is stronger and more powerful than the lines of communication found in the table of organization.

Good leaders and managers are aware of these informal communication patterns and they support the "grapevine" unless it is spreading rumors and misinformation, at which time the leader intervenes by providing correct and accurate information to reverse misinformation.

Collaboration with Other Departments

Although in most healthcare facilities there are separate risk management, quality management and infection control and prevention departments, this separation should not impede close cooperation and collaboration between the groups. These groups are closely aligned with the infection control program, its activities and sentinel event identification and reporting, as fully discussed above.

Regulatory Compliance

Infection control professionals must monitor compliance with all regulatory and recommending bodies in a continuous and ongoing monitoring. Some of these issues include structures, like policies, procedures and reporting systems; other issues include processes like a risk assessment and surveillance; still more relate to the outcomes of the infection control program and all of its activities.

PLANNING

CONDUCTING AN INFECTION RISK ASSESSMENT

The dynamic, systematic, goal-oriented problem solving approach to infection control consists of a five-phase cyclical process:

- *Assessment*: Data collection relating to the risks of infection

- *Identifying the Problem*: The collected data is organized and analyzed to identify and define health-related problems and concerns, like the risk of infection, and the strengths and weaknesses of the organization in terms of addressing these risks.

- *Planning*: Establishing priorities, developing expected outcomes of care, or goals, and selecting appropriate interventions to fulfill these goals.

- *Implementation:* The actual performance of interventions and the assessment of responses to interventions.

- *Evaluation:* Most similar to the assessment phase; it cycles right back into it. Data is collected relating to the current status as compared to the established expected outcomes. This conclusion reflects whether or not these goals were met. Should the interventions continue, be modified or ended because the goal has or has not been met?

THE PURPOSE OF RISK ASSESSMENTS

According to JCAHO, healthcare-associated infections and risks differ among facilities; therefore, control and prevention strategies must be tailored according to the organization's specific risk assessments.

Periodic risk assessments ensure that the organization is able to prevent and control infections from multidrug resistant organisms and from breaches, in terms of hand washing, standard and special contact precautions, cleaning, disinfection, sterilization, and other risks.

When the risk assessment reveals a deficiency, it is expected that the infection control professional educate staff about these risks and how to eliminate them, educate patients who are infected or colonized with resistant pathogens, educate family members about prevention, plan and implement a targeted, rather than organization-wide, surveillance program for resistant organisms as based on the risk assessment, and monitor and evaluate the outcomes that have resulted from these efforts.

Outcome evaluation data should minimally include, for example, quality information that reflects accurate resistant organism infection rates, the organization's compliance with external regulatory and recommending bodies, compliance with evidence based guidelines or best practices, the appropriateness and timeliness of intervention, compliance with the established laboratory based alert system that identifies new patients, transferred patients and readmitted patients affected with a multidrug resistant organisms, and the evaluation of all education activities given to staff, patients and significant others in terms of the effective and behavioral outcomes of that education.

MISSION, VISION AND VALUES

Infection prevention and control departments should have a written mission statement, vision statement, and set of values that are well thought out, formalized and documented.

MISSION STATEMENTS

Mission statements should be brief, yet broad, and should provide the basic foundation for the entire infection prevention and control department's vision, values, objectives, activities and action plans. These statements should motivate the members of the department with a shared perspective. The mission is the underlying framework of the department, which broadly describes everything about the organization or department and what is does. At times, goals, objectives, and the vision are also incorporated into the mission statement.

An example of a mission statement that can be used for an infection prevention and control department is, "To provide quality services that improve the levels of health and wellness for all the individuals we serve".

VISION STATEMENT

Vision Statements, like mission statements, are congruent with the department's mission and purpose, and they provide the department with basic values and beliefs. They give members of the department, and others in the organization, clear behavioral expectations.

VALUES

An organization should select core values that sum up their guiding moral principles. For example, here are CDC's stated values:

1. "Be a diligent steward of the funds entrusted to our agency

2. Provide an environment for intellectual and personal growth and integrity

3. Base all public health decisions on the highest quality scientific data that is derived openly and objectively

4. Place the benefits to society above the benefits to our institution

5. Treat all persons with dignity, honesty, and respect"

OBJECTIVES AND GOALS

Objectives and goals are specific statements used to plan and to evaluate infection control and prevention activities and the infection control program in its entirety.

The SMARTTA framework can be used for setting goals:

- S - Specific
- M - Measurable
- A - Achievable
- R - Realistic
- T - Timeframe
- T - Trackable
- A - Agreed to by the patient and significant other(s)

The CDC and JCAHO are useful resources for infection control professionals to use as a basis of the development of infection control and prevention department objectives and goals. The CDC's Healthy People Goals guide national health promotion and disease prevention efforts to improve the health of those in the United States. JCAHO establishes Patient Safety Goals on an annual basis.

SELECTING SUPPLIES, EQUIPMENT AND RESOURCES

SUPPLIES, EQUIPMENT AND RESOURCES

The infection control professional should have active participation in the selection of supplies and equipment for the infection control and prevention program. Some of these supplies and equipment are needed for the internal office functioning of the department and other supplies and equipment are related to patient care and infection prevention. For example, the infection control professional will want to investigate and recommend the purchase of software packages to track and trend infection related data, and they will also select care-related supplies and equipment like needleless systems.

Preventing Needlestick Injuries

According to NIOSH's Preventing Needlestick Injuries in Health Care Settings, the process used for the selection of and evaluation of safe needle devices requires that the infection control professional convene an interdisciplinary group that will collaboratively:

- Evaluate needle devices with safety features

- Conduct a product evaluation that includes the users of the device and the impact on the patient using clear criteria for measurement

- Educate healthcare workers about the correct, proper and safe use of the selected device

- Generate, implement and evaluate plans to reduce the number of sharps injuries in the facility.

- Perform risk assessments and post exposure assessment when injuries occur

- Establish priorities of action when assessments indicate the need for an action and an action plan

- Recognize that hollow bore needles have the greatest risk in terms of an occupational needle injury

HUMAN RESOURCES

The infection control and prevention department must have adequate staff to accomplish its mission, vision, goals and objectives. These numbers are based on a number of different factors and considerations, such as the size and complexity of the healthcare facility, the type of facility, the needs of the facility in terms of the intensity of its necessary infection control and prevention activities, and the ability of the organization to fund these salaries and benefits.

CONDUCTING EVALUATIONS

COST-BENEFIT ANALYSIS

Cost-benefit analysis compares and contrasts the benefits and costs associated with an intervention. This analysis moves beyond simply comparing two treatment options based on which one is less costly. In cost-benefit analysis, quantitative monetary value and the benefits to the patient are also analyzed. Infection control professionals use cost-benefit analysis to compare the costs of several treatments, as well as the benefits to the patient, and then decide which treatment or procedure is better suited for the specific patient. The cost-benefit analysis provides a justification for why a specific treatment or procedure is selected from all the alternatives.

3-E STUDIES

Efficacy, effectiveness and efficiency are similar and interconnected concepts, but there are key differences:

- *Efficacy*: the capacity or ability for something to produce the desired outcome under *ideal* circumstances.

- *Effectiveness*: the capacity or ability for something to produce the desired outcome under *real world* circumstances

- *Efficiency*: this describes the amount of resources needed for something to produce the desired outcome. When something is maximally efficient, it requires the least possible resources. When something is inefficient, it takes up more resources than it should.

Infection control and prevention departments and professionals should monitor and assess their programs' efficacy, effectiveness and efficiency. Additionally, opportunities for improvement should be identified and performance improvement interventions should be implemented.

RECOMMENDING CHANGES IN PRACTICE

Changes in practice should be recommended and implemented not only to correct deficiencies, but also to increase levels of performance to enhance clinical outcomes and save costs. All of these efforts can be accomplished with risk management and quality/performance improvement activities.

EDUCATION

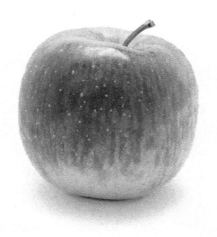

This section will provide you with the knowledge and skills to serve as an educator and researcher. You will learn how to assess educational needs, plan activities, implement programs and evaluate their outcomes in a number of different ways. You will also learn about the research process, how to apply critical thinking skills to research findings and how to incorporate research into practice.

HEALTH EDUCATION

In addition to empowerment and social marketing, health education is a highly important aspect of health promotion. Health education facilitates the individual's or group's ability to make knowledgeable decisions, and motivates behavioral change by influencing values and beliefs. The goals of health education include:

- The prevention of infection
- Increased patient and family coping
- Enhanced patient participation in decision making
- The development of self-care skills
- Increasing the potential for compliance with the health care regimen and health recommendations
- Adoption of healthier lifestyle choices
- Increased continuing care of ongoing, specific conditions

THE DOMAINS OF LEARNING

There are three domains of learning. These domains are the cognitive, psychomotor and affective domains.

- *The Cognitive Domain:* This domain consists of both knowledge and understanding. An example of a cognitive domain patient outcome is, "The patient verbalized knowledge of all of their medications and side effects". The six levels from the basic to the most complex are knowledge, comprehension, application, analysis, synthesis and evaluation. Some of the teaching/learning strategies for this domain include online/computer based learning, peer group discussions, reading material and a discussion or lecture.

- *The Psychomotor Domain:* The psychomotor domain consists of "hands-on skills" like taking blood pressure and using a blood glucose monitor correctly. The seven levels of this domain are perception, set, guided response, mechanism, complex overt response, adaptation and origination. Some of the teaching/learning strategies for this domain include demonstration, return demonstration and a video with a demonstration of the psychomotor skill.

- *The Affective Domain:* The affective domain includes the development of attitudes, beliefs, values and opinions. An example of affective domain competency is developing a belief that exercise is a valuable part of wellness. There are five levels are receiving, responding, valuing, organization and characterization by a value or a value complex. The teaching/learning strategies for this domain include role-playing and values clarification exercises. The affective domain is rarely used for patient teaching.

THE TEACHING PROCESS

ASSESSMENT

The purpose of assessment is to collect data about the learner(s) and their actual or potential learning needs. Within the community, the target group is identified and their learning needs are assessed. The assessment phase should include the identification of learning needs and the identification of influences that can impact on the learning process.

An assessment includes data about the learner (their current knowledge or skill, strengths and weaknesses, health beliefs, existing barriers to learning and behavior change, level of motivation, health problems, age related and cultural characteristics, as influencing factors in the learning process, preferences, learning style, etc.) and the learning need (What does the person know now? What should they know or be able to do?)

The assessment can be done using the dimensions model of community health as a framework.

The following dimensions are assessed and addressed:

- Biophysical
- Psychological
- Physical environment
- Sociocultural
- Behavioral
- Health services

PLANNING

The purpose of planning is to analyze the assessment data and come to some conclusion about the goals of the education, learning objectives, content to be addressed, strategies to meet these goals and a teaching plan that is consistent with the learning need(s) and the learner characteristics and preferences, including cultural beliefs, cultural practices, language and literacy, or health literacy, level. Planning consists of:

- Establishing priorities
- Determining and developing learning goals and objectives
- Selecting an appropriate teaching/learning strategy
- Selecting, organizing and developing content

IMPLEMENTATION

The purpose of implementation is to execute the teaching plan. Implementation may involve a lecture or using a videotape, for example.

EVALUATION

The purpose of evaluation is to determine whether or not the individual, or group, has met the pre-established learning objectives. Evaluation allows us to assess the teaching and learning processes and to determine its effects on the health of the learner.

Evaluation can be done by using a test or oral questioning (cognitive domain) or by asking the person to demonstrate a behavior or skill (psychomotor domain), depending on which domain of learning was addressed with the education.

BARRIERS TO LEARNING

LITERACY

Sadly, many Americans can't read at all. Some may only be able to read and comprehend material at a low-grade level. It is sometimes recommended that patient education material be authored at or below a sixth-grade reading level to accommodate for comprehension and literacy needs. You must assess the patient's literacy level and provide appropriate learning materials.

HEALTH LITERACY

Patients are considered "health literate" when they are able to understand information and use it to make appropriate health care decisions. Almost 50% of patients are NOT health literate. You must modify your communication and teaching to ensure comprehension. For example, simple anatomy and physiology information is preferable to complex, biochemical explanations that the patient cannot understand.

MOTIVATION AND READINESS

Patients will not learn unless they are motivated and ready to do so. You can motivate learners by involving them in the entire teaching/learning process, by focusing the learning on solving immediate and pressing concerns and by explaining the benefits of learning in terms of problem resolution, while maintaining an environment that is supportive of open, honest and respectful learning.

CULTURAL ASPECTS

Communication patterns, vocabulary, slang and terminology are differences that separate members of a group or culture, from others. You must become culturally competent about the norms and gestures of others, and modify terminology and behavior accordingly.

LANGUAGE BARRIERS

Communicating with and teaching those who speak a different language is challenging. However, these barriers can be overcome with some simple techniques such as speaking slowly, clarifying, re-clarifying, using pictures and diagrams, and eliciting the help of an interpreter.

HEALTH BELIEFS

Health beliefs can also be a barrier to learning and changes in behavior. Patients who place a high value on health, health promotion and wellness will be more highly motivated to learn. You can overcome health belief-related barriers by facilitating the patient's understanding of the importance of these values in concrete terms that promotes their health.

PSYCHOLOGICAL FACTORS

Healthcare professionals have to assess and accommodate for any actual or potential cognitive, sensory and psychological/emotional barriers to learning. For example, cognitive limitations can be overcome with slow, brief, simple and understandable explanations. Psychological barriers can be minimized by establishing trust, reinforcing learning with positive feedback, and minimizing stress.

PHYSICAL CAPABILITIES AND LIMITATIONS

Sensory barriers can be accommodated for with large print materials and Braille for the visually impaired, louder discussions with patients affected with a hearing loss, and the use of assistive devices like magnifiers, eyeglasses and hearing aids. Functional limitations can also impede learning.

LEARNER CHARACTERISTICS

Some of the unique characteristics of learners include their individual learning style and preferences, cultural impacts, literacy, health literacy and level of motivation and readiness.

DEVELOPING MEASURABLE GOALS AND OBJECTIVES

Learning objectives guide the teaching process and enable us to objectively evaluate outcomes and effectiveness. Learning objectives are established during the planning phase of the patient and family education process.

Learning goals are statements regarding the expected behavior change that the teaching episode should facilitate. For example, a goal may be practicing safe sex practices.

Learning objectives, or outcomes, reflect what the person will know, or do, during and after the teaching episode. These objectives or outcomes reflect the steps that the person must do, or know, in order to reach the ultimate goal. For example, the person should be able to discuss various sexually transmitted diseases or how unsafe sexual practices increase a person's risk to them. These objectives enable the person to achieve their learning goal. Learning objectives must be:

- Learner, not teacher oriented
- Specific
- Measurable and behavioral
- Congruent with the domain and level of knowledge
- Consistent with the assessed need

The table on the next page shows desirable objectives on the left, and undesirable objectives on the right:

Appropriate LOs	Inappropriate LOs
Learner Oriented: **The learner will be able to describe proper hand washing.**	Teacher-Oriented: The healthcare professional will instruct the patient about proper hand washing.
Specific: **The learner will be able to list the steps of hand washing.**	Non-Specific: The learner will be able to discuss hand washing.
Measurable/ Behavioral: **The learner will correctly demonstrate proper hand washing.**	Non Measurable & Non Behavioral: The learner will be able to understand hand washing.
Consistent With Learning Domain: **The learner will be able to demonstrate proper hand washing procedure.**	Inconsistent With Learning Domain: The learner will be able to describe the proper hand washing procedure.
Consistent With Level of Domain: **Categorize the degree of risk associated with multiple & complex relationships (synthesis)**	Inconsistent With Level of Domain: List (knowledge) the degree of risk associated with multiple & complex risk factor relationships (synthesis)

The best way to write learning objectives is to begin the learning objective with the statement, "At the conclusion of the teaching, the learner will be able to:" and then start the statement with a measurable verb that is consistent with the domain of learning.

DEVELOPING A TEACHING PLAN

THE SEQUENCING OF INFORMATION

Generally speaking, content and information should be sequenced from the known to the unknown, from the simple to the complex and from the least threatening to the most threatening.

For example, when the infection control professional wants to teach about the chain of infection, the educator will sequence the content and information to move the patient from information about the basic ways that infections can be spread (simple and known) to the characteristics of a susceptible host (complex and unknown). Additionally, when teaching the patient about changing a surgical dressing, the educator will allow the patient to practice dressing techniques on a medical model (less threatening) and then move the patient to change their own abdominal dressing (more threatening).

The knowledge, skills and abilities will also be sequenced according to the levels of complexity for each of the domains of learning.

Teaching strategies must be selected based on the domain of learning that is being taught. For example, lecture and discussion are appropriate strategies for the cognitive domain and demonstration, return demonstration and practice are appropriate strategies for the psychomotor domain.

Content is also developed in order to ensure that it is current, accurate and appropriate to the learning need.

Sample Teaching Plan (Curriculum)

TITLE: Medical-Surgical Asepsis and Infection Control
DURATION: 2 hours
METHOD OF EVALUATION: 20 Question Multiple Choice Quiz

LEARNING OBJECTIVES	CONTENT	TIME	METHODOLOGY
1. Define asepsis, differentiate medical/surgical asepsis, and differentiate cleaning, disinfection and sterilization.	**Definitions** - Asepsis - Sepsis - Microorganisms - Pathogens - Infection Control **Medical Asepsis** - Definition - Examples **Surgical Asepsis** - Definition - Examples **Cleaning** - Definition - Examples **Disinfection** - Definition - Examples **Sterilization** - Definition - Examples	5 mins	Lecture and Discussion

2. Detail the chain of infection	**Causative Agent** • Definition • Examples **The Reservoir** • Definition • Examples **Portal of Exit** • Definition • Examples **Method of Trans-mission** • Definition • Examples **Portal of Entry** • Definition • Examples **Susceptible Host** • Definition • Examples	10 mins	Lecture and Discussion

3. List and describe different types of micro-organisms and the types of infection.	**Bacteria** • Aerobic and Anaerobic • Examples • Primary Reservoir • Type of Infection **Viruses** • RNA and DNA • Examples • Primary Reservoir • Type of Infection **Fungi** • Examples • Primary Reservoir • Type of Infection **Parasites** • Examples • Primary Reservoir • Type of Infection **Protozoa** • Examples • Primary Reservoir • Type of Infection **Infections** • Acute • Chronic • Local • Systemic • Bacteremia • Septicemia	10 mins	Lecture and Discussion

APPLYING THE PRINCIPLES OF ADULT LEARNING

Andragogy, or adult learning, has immediate usefulness in terms of solving problems; it involves active learner involvement and participation; curriculum and content are based on the learner's needs and desires. Below is a table that compares and contrasts pedagogy and andragogy.

	Pedagogy	**Andragogy**
Curriculum	The state and the teacher develop and design the teaching, based on what they decide is important.	The learner, in collaboration with the diabetes educator, develops and designs the teaching, based on learner needs and characteristics, such as their preferred learning style.
Level of Input	The child is a somewhat passive learner. The learner has a low level of involvement in all the phases of the teaching process.	The adult is a highly active learner. The learner has a high level of involvement in all the phases of the teaching process.
Teaching Methods	Homework & Teacher Lecture	Active learner participation The adult learner has a large amount of knowledge and experiences to share with others and to relate to the learning activity.
Purpose of Learning	Childhood learning has little immediate application. This learning prepares the child for the future and their future needs.	Adult learning should have immediate application and usefulness. The learning aims to solve problems.

LENGTH/DURATION OF THE TEACHING SESSION

Even the most experienced educators can have problems accurately planning the duration of a teaching session. The reason for this is because there are a number of factors that can affect the amount of time needed to effectively facilitate learning. There are some general principles, however, that should be considered when planning for teaching/learning interaction. They are as follows:

A psychomotor need is best met with short teaching sessions for each step of the procedure or process. This principle is applied to teaching, relating to things like foot care and dressing changes for a wound. The educator should allow the patient ample time in between sessions so the patient can practice without the stress of another's presence, particularly when the learner is affected with a physical or functional impairment.

Short-term memory decreases as a function of the natural aging process. Repetition and hence, more time, may be necessary for the aging patient and/or family member(s).

Children, the cognitively impaired and those with a serious illness and/or pain have a short attention span. Teaching/learning sessions for these patients and family members should be brief and modified, as based on the individual's need.

Learning is often best accomplished with short sessions over time, when time permits. For example, a cognitive need, such as the need to learn about discharge instructions, is best accomplished with a brief session about the medications the patient will take when discharged and then another session, on the following day, that teaches the patient about community resources that could benefit them.

Heterogeneous (mixed groups of varying knowledge) and large groups tend to require more time for a teaching session than homogeneous (similar group members in terms of knowledge) or smaller groups.

EVALUATING LEARNER OUTCOMES

There are two types of evaluation in the teaching/learning process. They are referred to as formative and summative evaluation.

FORMATIVE EVALUATION

Formative evaluation is defined as the continuous assessment of how effective the learning is during the time that the learning activity is actually being implemented.

The purpose of formative evaluation is to allow us to modify the established teaching plan if, during the course of the learning activity, it does not appear that the outcomes are being successfully achieved. For example, if the teaching plan consisted of a videotape about the need for immunizations, and the learner is not able to capture the concepts surrounding the mode of transmission, it may be necessary to alter the plan and have, instead, a brief discussion about the modes of transmission that is then followed with the discussion or some printed material. Then, on the next day, you will proceed with the established teaching plan.

If the formative evaluation is unsatisfactory, consider whether:

- There are any learning barriers the plan did not assess or consider
- The time allocation is adequate
- The reading material is at the appropriate grade level of reading
- The environment is conducive to learning
- The learner is committed to the learning objectives
- The learning objectives were realistic
- The teaching methodology is appropriate

SUMMATIVE EVALUATION

Summative evaluation allows us to determine whether or not the education has achieved the established learning objectives for the individual or group. Did the learning activity successfully close the gap between what should be and what actually is?

Education can be deemed effective when the pre-established learning objectives are achieved. When one or more learning objectives have not been achieved, the education has not been effective and, therefore, the teacher must return to the assessment phase of the process to validate the accuracy of assessed needs, then to the planning phase to determine whether or not this phase is educationally sound and then make any necessary modifications needed to achieve desired outcomes during future re-teaching sessions.

Evaluation is more than a survey that asks how the learner felt about the room, the teacher and their satisfaction with the educational activity. Evaluation consists of comparing the outcome knowledge, or skill, to the established learning objective. If it does, the teaching has been effective. If it does NOT match the pre-established learning objective, the activity was ineffective and the process must be repeated.

Remember that learning is not always permanent. It is important for health care providers to periodically assess the patient to determine if the knowledge or skill has been retained over time. Learning reinforcement is necessary when the knowledge or skill has not been retained.

Immediate Summative Evaluation

Immediate summative evaluation strategies that are appropriate for each of the domains include:

Cognitive Domain	Psychomotor Domain	Affective Domain
• **Oral Questioning** • **Written Tests**	• Return Demonstration	• Changed Belief, Attitude or Value

Long Term Summative Evaluation

- Has the patient, family member or the group retained the learning over time?

- Did the patient, or patient population, call the physician when they experienced a suspected adverse drug reaction to their antibiotic?

- Has the number of readmissions secondary to surgical wound infections decreased after education about wound care and sterile dressing changes?

- Has the number of pediatric patients receiving immunizations increased?

- Has the education been effective in decreasing lengths of stay for resistant pathogen affected patients?

- Has the education decreased the rate of postoperative pneumonia within the facility?

- Has the patient/family teaching decreased the number and frequency of unexpected returns to the emergency room or the primary physician?

- Have community, group and individual educational endeavors increased customer satisfaction scores?

The answers to these questions reflect the true purpose of education - a change in behavior. A change in behavior should be measurable for both individuals and groups. These changes in behavior are the true outcomes of education.

Furthermore, when a patient teaching plan has been successful, it is advisable to accept and adopt it as the standard for the entire facility in order to ensure that there is no variation in process and that successful outcomes can be maintained and predictable throughout the organization. For example, if the preoperative teaching class for elderly patients has a correlation with decreased rates of hospital-acquired pneumonia, this class should be replicated without variation to perpetuate this success with other learners.

INFECTION PREVENTION AND CONTROL EDUCATION

The components of a teaching plan for patients, family members and visitors about ways to prevent and control infections vary somewhat among groups. For example, visitors may have to be taught only about hand-washing, the donning of personal protective equipment, and special isolation precautions; however, patient/family teaching should be more comprehensive. Some of the components of a teaching plan for patients, family members can include, among others, the following, as based on the patient and family's assessed educational needs:

- Asepsis: Medical and Surgical Asepsis
- Hand-washing
- The Chain of Infection
- Special Precautions
- Protective Measures Such as Personal Protective Equipment and Immunizations
- Antibiotics: Use, Dosage, Side Effects, Adverse Reactions and Compliance

EDUCATION RESEARCH

EDUCATION RESEARCH EVALUATION - OVERVIEW

There are many areas of healthcare education that can and should be evaluated with formal and informal research activities. For example, you could evaluate the structures, the processes and the outcomes; you can evaluate individual educational offerings or you could research your overall educational program; you can also research and evaluate individual educational activities and/or the overall educational program in terms of things like learner satisfaction, cost avoidance, and other potential benefits like decreased rates of hospitalization, self-care abilities and active participation in health promotion and preventive health, for example.

A through critique of research includes all the steps of a research project and all elements of the research report. These areas of consideration for the research critique are as follows:

- Title
- Abstract
- Introduction
- Review of the literature
- Methodology
- Data analysis
- Discussion of the research findings

- Summary
- Conclusion
- Implications
- Recommendations
- Ethical considerations
- Biases

GENERAL CONSIDERATIONS

Is the research study complete, objective, concise and presented in an understandable and logical manner?

- Are the tables, charts and graphs labeled and understandable?

- Are the references appropriate and current?
- Is the research study significant in terms of infection control?
- What are the overall strengths of the research project?
- What are the overall weaknesses of the research project?
- Are the findings valid and useful to other healthcare professionals?
- Are the author's claims substantiated?

CRITIQUING QUANTITATIVE RESEARCH

TITLE

- Is the title brief?
- Does the title accurately reflect the study, and the purpose of the study?
- Does it reflect the variables and the population?

ABSTRACT

- Does the abstract reflect the purpose of the study and its significance?
- Does it include the research methodology and information about the sample and the sample selection process?
- Does the abstract include the conclusions and interpretation of the findings?

INTRODUCTION

- Is the purpose of the study clearly identified?
- Is the problem statement included in the introduction?

- Is the significance of the study included in the introduction?
- What is the significance of the study?
- What possible benefits can be derived from this study?
- Are operational definitions included?
- Are the assumptions and delimitations stated?
- Does the introduction reflect possible practical applications?
- Is the hypothesis, or hypotheses, included in the introduction?
- Are the conceptual framework and its appropriateness included in the introduction?
- Is the introduction brief, logical and understandable?

REVIEW OF LITERATURE

- Are all relevant sources included?
- Are the sources current (< 5 years) unless they have historical value?
- Are primary sources used when appropriate?
- Are empirical research studies included in the review of the literature?
- Did it give you in-depth information and a fuller understanding of the topic of interest?
- Did the researcher obtain and relate information about the design the study in terms of methodology, variables, concepts, subjects, sampling, and data analysis, among other things?
- Is the review of the literature organized, objective and without bias?
- Is the bibliography or reference list complete and appropriate?
- Is there a reference for every citation made in the text?

METHODOLOGY

- Is the research design (methodology) clearly identified?
- Was this methodology appropriate for this research study?
- Does it detail how the study was conducted?
- Does it clearly state how the data was analyzed?
- Was the data analyzed in the appropriate and accurate manner?
- Is the setting for the research clearly stated and appropriate to the study?
- Is the type of sample appropriate for this research study?
- Is this method of sampling appropriate for this research study?
- Was the sample large enough for the study?
- Were the subjects representative of the population?
- Were criteria for inclusion and exclusion of subjects stated and valid?
- Did the research study clearly indicate what kind or method of measurement and measurement tools were used?
- Did it include a copy of the measurement instrument that was used?
- Did the research study include statements about the validity and reliability of the measurement instrument that was used?
- Was the validity of this instrument sufficient for the study?
- Was the reliability of this instrument sufficient for the study?
- Are the data collection methods or interventions used for the study clearly stated and sound?
- Is the data collection organized?
- Is the procedure for the data collection methods or interventions clearly stated?

DATA ANALYSIS

- What type of data analysis was used?
- Is the statistical analysis method appropriate for the data and the study?
- Was the analysis mathematically accurate?
- Did the analysis support or refute the alternative hypothesis or hypotheses?

DISCUSSION OF THE RESEARCH FINDINGS

- Is the presentation and interpretation of the research findings logical, organized and cogent?
- Is the discussion of the research findings complete?
- Does the discussion of the research findings address cautions relating to the generalizing the findings to other populations?

SUMMARY

- Is the summary brief and concise?
- Does the summary include a brief statement about the purpose of the study?
- Does the summary include a brief statement about assumptions that underlie the study?
- Does the summary include a brief statement about the how the hypotheses were tested?
- What other things should have been included in the summary that were not included?

CONCLUSIONS

- Are the conclusions summarized in a logical, brief and cogent manner?
- Is the summary of data analysis relating to the null hypothesis and other hypotheses presented in a complete, accurate and understandable manner?

IMPLICATIONS OF THE STUDY

- Do the implications relate to and benefit health education?
- Is there an emphasis on the importance of this study?

RECOMMENDATIONS

- Are the recommendations consistent with the results of the research findings?
- Are these recommendations valid and accurate, based on the research study?

ETHICAL CONSIDERATIONS

- Were all ethical rights and principles upheld?

BIAS

- Was sample selection, measurement, response, procedural and researcher bias present and acknowledged by the researcher(s)?

CRITIQUING QUALITATIVE RESEARCH

PHILOSOPHICAL OR THEORETICAL SOUNDNESS

- Are the findings developed and clearly expressed?

- Are the findings logically consistent and compatible with the knowledge base of health education?

- Are the assumptions and methodological procedures consistent and compatible with the philosophical or theoretical basis of the study?

- Are the data analytic approaches and data interpretation consistent and compatible with the philosophical or theoretical basis of the study?

METHODOLOGICAL CONSISTENCY AND CONGRUENCE

- Is there adequate documentation supporting the rationale for selection of the participants, the context, and location of the study?

- Are any threats to validity acknowledged?

- Did the researcher scrupulously adhere to the established procedures?

DESCRIPTIVE VIVIDNESS

- Did the researcher include essential descriptive information in a clear and understandable manner?

- Are adequate interpretative and analytic skills demonstrated in the description of the phenomenon of interest?

ANALYSIS PRECISION

- Does the analysis accurately interpret the data?

INTERPRETATION PRECISION

- Did the outcome of the study give meaning to the phenomenon under study?
- Did the researcher present a meaningful and precise picture of the phenomenon under study?

HEURISTIC RELEVANCE

- Did the researcher clearly present the phenomenon?
- Did the researcher clearly present the applicability of the study to health education?
- Were you able to readily recognize the phenomenon and its connection to you, as a health educator and the profession of health education?
- What new knowledge was gained as a result of this study?

PUTTING FINDINGS INTO PRACTICE

There are many areas of healthcare education that can and should be evaluated with formal and informal research activities. For example, you could evaluate the structures, the processes and the outcomes; you can evaluate individual educational offerings or you could research your overall educational program; you can also research and evaluate individual educational activities and/or the overall educational program in terms of things like learner satisfaction, cost avoidance, and other potential benefits like decreased rates of hospitalization, self-care abilities and active participation in health promotion and preventive health, for example.

In terms of infection control and prevention practices, evidence based practices and best practices can, and should be integrated into practice, educational activities and consultative actions. The application of evidence based practices and best practices were fully discussed and described above.

PRACTICE EXAMINATION

MULTIPLE-CHOICE QUIZ

1. Which professional organization certifies those who practice in infection control and epidemiology?

A. The Centers for Disease Control and Prevention

B. The American Certification Board of Infection Control and Epidemiology

C. The Association of Infection Control and Epidemiology Certification

D. The Certification Board of Infection Control and Epidemiology

2. Which body accredits the Certification Board of Infection Control and Epidemiology?

A. The Centers for Disease Control and Prevention

B. The National Commission on Certifying Agencies

C. The Association of Infection Control and Epidemiology Certification

D. The Joint Commission on the Accreditation of Healthcare Organizations

3. Which governmental agency provides the most regulations and guidelines for infection control and prevention?

A. The U.S. Occupational and Safety and Health Administration

B. Association for Professionals in Infection Control and Epidemiology

C. The Centers for Disease Control and Prevention

D. The Joint Commission on the Accreditation of Healthcare Organizations

4. **What is the primary and ultimate purpose of infection surveillance?**

A. To fulfill the requirements of external regulatory agencies

B. To identify problems in terms of infection control and prevention

C. To determine current and projected morbidity and mortality rates

D. To develop and implement corrective action and improvement plans

5. **Risk stratification is a technique used in which type of study or investigation?**

A. A risk assessment

B. An epidemiologic study

C. A qualitative study

D. A quantitative study

6. **Which standard of practice and role for the infection control and prevention professional requires that this professional provide expert knowledge and guidance to others?**

A. Consultation

B. Advocacy

C. Collaboration

D. Assessment

7. Specific standardized terms and terminology are used in infection control and prevention in order to:

A. Facilitate consistent communication for reporting and other purposes

B. Enable the patient to understand more fully infections and prevention

C. Help the members of the healthcare facility to comply with policies

D. Provide a deeper knowledge of infections and infection prevention

8. Select the term that is accurately paired with its definition in terms of transmission.

A. Vehicle Transmission: Infections spread with vehicles like ticks

B. Vector Transmission: Infections spread with inanimate objects

C. Airborne Transmission: The pathogen is inhaled as a droplet nuclei

D. Direct Contact Transmission: The host has contact with a contaminated inanimate object.

9. You are working with a group of clinicians to explore newer and safer products, such as needleless systems, to decrease the rate of occupational exposures. Why are you, according to law, involving others like nurses and physicians, in making these selection decisions?

A. It is legally mandated to do so.

B. It is recommended to do so.

C. Change will be more accepted.

D. Collective decisions are better than singular decisions.

10. A needleless system is considered what kind of control?

A. A work practice control.

B. An administrative control.

C. An engineering control.

D. A preventive control.

11. You have just written a policy and procedure relating to the cleaning of reusable supplies and equipment. Which of the following is the best statement to include in this policy and procedure in terms of the purpose of cleaning?

A. The purpose of cleaning is to ensure that the items are medically aseptic.

B. The purpose of cleaning is to ensure that the items are surgically aseptic.

C. The purpose of cleaning is to ensure that the items are aseptic.

D. The purpose of cleaning is to ensure adequate and complete disinfection.

12. The primary difference between colonization and infection is that colonization...

A. Varies according to the person's immune responses

B. Can be detected by the laboratory and infection cannot be detected.

C. Occurs only as the result of microorganisms not capable of leading to infection.

D. Is the presence of microorganisms on bodily surfaces that do not cause disease or symptoms.

13. The chain of infection in correct sequential order is the:

A. The agent, the reservoir, the environment, the mode of transmission, the portal of entry, the portal of exit and the susceptible host.

B. The reservoir, the agent, the environment, the mode of transmission, the portal of entry, the portal of exit and the susceptible host.

C. The reservoir, the environment, the agent, the mode of transmission, the portal of entry, the portal of exit and the susceptible host.

D. The reservoir, the mode of transmission, the environment, the agent, the portal of entry, the portal of exit and the susceptible host.

14. Which of the following is a factor intrinsic to the pathogen that affects the ability of a pathogenic microorganism to cause disease?

A. The susceptibility of the host

B. Its virulence

C. Its mode of transmission

D. The immune status of the host

15. Select the term accurately paired with its description.

A. Pathogenicity: The ratio of those who develop the infection compared to the number exposed to it

B. Virulence: The number of pathogens in a colony

C. Infective dose: The established 60% dose that leads to infection

D. Assimilation: How well the pathogen adjusts to its environment

16. Which of the following infections is caused by a rod shaped bacteria?

A. Syphilis

B. Candida albicans

C. Tuberculosis

D. HIV

17. Gram negative bacteria:

A. React to the gram stain.

B. Are less common than gram positive bacteria.

C. Have thicker cell walls than gram positive bacteria.

D. Include salmonella and shigella.

18. Your patient is affected with M. Tuberculosis mycobacteria. What would you most likely expect to see in terms of the patient's microbiology laboratory findings?

A. A change in color when stained with the Ziehl-Neelsen stain

B. A change in color when stained with the Kinyoun stain

C. No change in color when stained with the Ziehl-Neelsen stain

D. No change in color when stained with Mercurium

19. The four phases of bacterial growth in correct and accurate sequential order are:

A. The lag phase, the log phase, the stationary phase and the death phase.

B. The log phase, the lag phase, the stationary phase and the death phase.

C. The lag phase, the genesis phase, the stationary phase and the death phase.

D. The genesis phase, the log phase, the stationary phase and the death phase.

20. Select the phase of bacterial growth that is accurately paired with its characteristic.

A. The Stationary Phase: Growth and metabolic activity decreases

B. The Death Phase: The bacteria is not acclimating to its new environment

C. The Lag Phase: The bacteria is without any nutrients at all

D. The Log Phase: The growth rate slows down

21. The stages of virus growth in correct sequential order include:

A. Attachment, un-coating, penetration, replication, self-assembly and release.

B. Attachment, penetration, un-coating, replication, self-assembly and release.

C. Attachment, replication, self-assembly penetration, un-coating and release.

D. Attachment, penetration, replication, un-coating, self-assembly and release.

22. Select the phase of bacterial growth accurately paired with its characteristic.

A. The Attachment Stage: The virus enters the host's cells

B. The Penetration Stage: The virus attaches to a receptor on the host's cellular surface

C. The Un-coating Stage: The viral capsid is removed, which allows its nucleic material to enter the bodily cells

D. The Un-coating Stage: The viral capsid is hardened, which allows its nucleic material to enter the bodily cells.

23. Which statement about fungi is true?

A. The vast majority of fungi are capable of leading to severe infections.

B. Fungi are classified as gram positive and gram negative.

C. Fungi have synergistic, antagonist, and commensal symbiotic relationships.

D. Symbiotic relationships benefit both the virus and the organism it attaches to.

24. Select the type of fungal infection accurately paired with its description.

A. Gram positive fungi react to a gram stain.

B. Acid fast fungi turn blue with the Ziehl-Neelsen stain.

C. Superficial fungal infections can affect the nails.

D. Aspergillosis can lead to a systemic fungal infection.

25. Select the parasitic infection that is accurately paired with its treatment.

A. Maggot infestation: Permethrin 5 percent, ivermectin, lindane, and crotamiton

B. Scabies: Ivermectin

C. Giardia: Metronidazole, tinidazole and nitazoxanide

D. Tapeworms: Penicillin and isolation

26. Your patient is affected with Lyme disease. This patient asks you how this infection was transmitted to him. What should your response be?

A. "You got it with direct transmission from a tick."

B. "You got it with direct transmission from a mosquito."

C. "You got it with vector transmission from a tick."

D. "You got it with vector transmission from a mosquito."

27. Which susceptible host is at greatest risk for an infection?

A. An immunosuppressed host who is exposed to a pathogen with high virulence and pathogenicity

B. An 84 year-old patient taking radiation therapy who is exposed to a fungus

C. A neonate who is exposed to a moderately virulent pathogen

D. A patient with a poor nutritional status and high levels of stress

28. Which is a nonspecific bodily defense against infection?

A. Antibody mediated defenses

B. Cell mediated defenses

C. Active immunity

D. The inflammatory process

29. An example of active, artificial immunity is:

A. The immunity that the newborn has at the time of birth.

B. Immunity that is acquired after having had the infection.

C. The immunity that is acquired after having had the flu vaccine.

D. The immunity that is acquired after having had immune globulin.

30. Select the level of prevention paired with its description.

A. Quaternary prevention: The focus on the prevention of any occurrence of disease

B. Primary prevention: Screening

C. Tertiary prevention: Restoration of function

D. Secondary prevention: Monitoring compliance with quarantine

31. You are teaching your patient's visitors about the proper donning of a gown and gloves. What domain of learning are you teaching?

A. Diabetes education

B. Cognitive

C. Affective

D. Psychomotor

32. Which teaching strategy is most appropriate when teaching a patient's visitors about properly donning a gown and gloves?

A. Discussion

B. Demonstration

C. Reading material

D. Role playing

33. Which is an appropriate expected outcome for an educational activity relating to changing a sterile surgical dressing?

A. The nurse will demonstrate how to properly change a dressing

B. The nurse will discuss how to properly change a dressing

C. The patient will demonstrate how to properly change a dressing

D. The patient will discuss how to properly change a dressing

34. Which best describes the application of research to practice?

A. Benchmarking practice

B. Evidence based practice

C. Professional critical thinking

D. Research analysis

35. You give a quiz to nurses after annual training about resistant pathogens. What type of educational evaluation is this?

  A. Formative evaluation

  B. Knowledge evaluation

  C. Interim evaluation

  D. Summative evaluation

36. Educational content should be sequenced from the:

  A. Threatening to non-threatening.

  B. Psychomotor to the cognitive domain.

  C. Unknown to the known.

  D. Simple to the complex.

37. Although risk management is closely aligned with continuous quality improvement, it differs in that it:

  A. Proactively addresses opportunities for improvement.

  B. Aims to reduce legal liability.

  C. Retroactively addresses opportunities for improvement.

  D. Is not required by JCAHO as continuous improvement is.

38. Root cause analysis can successfully find:

  A. Which individual made a mistake

  B. Which people made a mistake

  C. Why nosocomial infections occur

  D. Problematic processes

39. What is the term that describes an occurrence that leads to, or has the potential to lead to, an adverse outcome?

   A. An adverse event

   B. A cardinal event

   C. A sentinel event

   D. A systemic variance

40. The infection control professional is doing a quality assurance/improvement study and notices that variance is occurring because of things inherent to the process. What kind of variance is this?

A. An independent variance

B. A dependent variance

C. A random variance

D. A specific variance

41. You are reading an infection control surveillance report and it states that the number of new influenza infections is 2: 1,000. What type of occurrence does this signify?

A. The rate of the infection

B. The incidence of the infection

C. The prevalence of the infection

D. The morbidity rate of the infection

42. **Over the last decade, the rate of influenza during the winter months in your local community has remained relatively stable, however, this year these rates of occurrence have doubled. How would you describe this event and situation?**

A. As a pandemic

B. As an epidemic

C. As endemic

D. As syndemic

43. **Which statement about incubation periods is accurate?**

A. The latent period is always longer than the incubation period.

B. The latent period and the incubation period are identical and synonymous.

C. The incubation period is the time between infection and the onset of symptoms.

D. The incubation period is the time between infection and infectiousness.

44. **The stages of infection in correct sequential order are the:**

A. Prodromal stage, the incubation stage, the illness stage and the convalescence stage.

B. Incubation stage, the illness stage, the prodromal stages and the convalescence stage.

C. Incubation stage, the preemptive stage, the illness stage and the convalescence stage.

D. Incubation stage, the prodromal stage, the illness stage and the convalescence stage.

45. Which stage of the infection process begins when symptoms begin and ends when the symptoms have disappeared?

A. The predromal stage

B. The prodromal stage

C. The illness stage

D. The preemptive stage

46. Which of the following is NOT one of the five classical signs and symptoms of a local infection?

A. Swelling

B. Heat

C. Malaise

D. Redness

47. Your female patient's laboratory test results have just been delivered to the patient care unit. This patient's erythrocyte sedimentation rate is 10 millimeters per hour, her C reactive protein is 8 mg/L, and her blood viscosity is 3 × 10□3. What would you suspect?

A. The absence of infection

B. The presence of a mild infection

C. The presence of a moderate infection

D. The presence of a severe infection

48. Which of the following values is a normal value for cerebrospinal fluid?

A. A pressure of 60 mm H20

B. A light yellow, clear appearance

C. 50 mg/100 mL of total protein

D. 90 mg/100 mL glucose

49. You are conducting an epidemiologic study using a measurement tool and a number of different data collectors. You soon notice that different data collection staff are scoring the same infection with different values. What should you be concerned about?

A. The validity of the measurement tool

B. The reliability of the measurement tool

C. The sensitivity of the measurement tool

D. The bias of the measurement tool

50. Select the antibiotic accurately paired with its pharmacological classification.

A. Vancomycin: Glycopeptides

B. Doripenem: Amsamycins

C. Clindamysin: Carbapenems

D. Erythromycin: Lincosamides

51. Select the antifungal drug accurately paired with its pharmacological classification.

A. Polyene antifungal drugs: Nafifine

B. Azole antifungal drugs: Fluconazole

C. Allylamine antifungal drugs: 5-Fluorocytosine

D. Antimetabolite antifungal drugs: Amphotericin

52. When is antimicrobial prophylaxis indicated?

A. Preoperatively before high risk procedures

B. Prior to the insertion of an indwelling urinary catheter

C. Prior to the insertion of an central venous catheter

D. Never, because it leads to resistant bacteria

53. Antimicrobials should be used based on infection site, host, and when possible, definitive diagnosis of the infection and offending pathogen. What type is not based on any of the above, but is still sometimes indicated?

A. Therapeutic use

B. Prophylactic use

C. Empiric use

D. Tentative use

54. Which age group is most at risk for otitis media?

A. Infants

B. School age children

C. Adolescents

D. Young adults

55. Which factor most commonly affects the frequency of infections among children who attend school?

A. An incomplete immunization history

B. The lack of immunizations

C. Poor hand washing

D. Coughing and sneezing

56. The design of a good surveillance program should include:

A. A review of the literature

B. Stakeholder involvement

C. The design of the study

D. Data analysis

57. Which of the following classifications is helpful for preserving the privacy and confidentiality of data obtained during surveillance studies?

A. The College of American Pathologists' Systematized Nomenclature of Medicine Classification

B. HIPPA's Security Rule Classification

C. The National Modifiable Disease Surveillance System Classification

D. HIPPA's Privacy Rule Classification

58. As you are about to disseminate the findings of your surveillance activities over the last year, what legal aspect must be ensured?

A. The validity of the data

B. The reliability of the data

C. The rights to privacy

D. The rights to autonomy

59. The CDC recommends that all infection control breaches are investigated in terms of:

A. The nature of the breach

B. The pathogen's prevalence

C. The pathogen's virulence

D. The pervasiveness of the pathogen

60. You have just discovered that the wrong procedures were used for the disinfection and sterilization of endoscopic equipment. What category of infection control breach is this?

A. Category A breach

B. Category B breach

C. A critical breach

D. A noncritical breach

61. Which category of infection control breach will most likely be reported to the affected patients?

A. Category A breach

B. Category B breach

C. Category C breach

D. None

62. Which fact about hepatitis B and/or hepatitis C is accurate?

A. Hepatitis B can be asymptomatic for up to 3 months and hepatitis C can be asymptomatic up to 2 months

B. Hepatitis C can be asymptomatic for up to 3 months and hepatitis B can be asymptomatic up to 2 months

C. Both hepatitis B and hepatitis C can both be asymptomatic for up to 3 months

D. Both hepatitis B and hepatitis C can both be asymptomatic for up to 6 months

63. Which statement about differentiating the acute and chronic forms of hepatitis B and/or hepatitis C is accurate?

A. The acute and chronic forms of hepatitis B can be differentiated with serologic tests.

B. The acute and chronic forms of hepatitis C can be differentiated with serologic tests.

C. The acute and chronic forms of hepatitis B and C can be differentiated with serologic tests.

D. The acute and chronic forms of hepatitis B and C cannot be differentiated with serologic tests.

64. Select the epidemiological term paired with its description:

A. Prevalence is an epidemiological statistic that tells us how virulent and powerful the pathogen is.

B. Incidence is the number of newly diagnosed cases in a specific population during a defined period of time.

C. Rate is calculated by dividing the number of new cases by the number of people in the risk population.

D. Morbidity rates tell us about the rates of death related to a specific infection or disease.

65. Which is the most accurate definition of risk?

A. Risk is the statistical significance of exposure.

B. Risk reflects genetic factors that can lead to illness.

C. Risk reflects the probability of getting a disease.

D. Risk reflects poor life style choices.

66. You have identified adolescents at greatest risk for a certain infection after having completed an in-depth surveillance study in the community. What is this group referred to as?

A. A target group, because they should be separated from the general population

B. A target group, because they should be provided with targeted interventions

C. A healthy group that is more at risk than others for this certain infection

D. A group that is more at risk than others and needs prophylactic antibiotics

67. Select the Component of Wellness that is accurately paired with its description.

A. Low level of susceptibility: A highly functioning immune system

B. High level of resilience: A highly functioning immune system

C. Emotional risk factor: Lack of insight

D. Economic risk factor: Occupational exposures

68. Your patient has expressed despair and a loss of meaning to their life. Which Component of Wellness places this patient at risk for diseases and illnesses?

A. Social risk factors

B. Psychological risk factors

C. Cultural risk factors

D. Spiritual risk factors

69. Which kind of epidemiological rate is most useful when interpreting data within context?

A. Crude rates

B. Adjusted rates

C. Morbidity rates

D. Mortality rates

70. Select the mortality rate that is accurately paired with its definition or description:

A. Neonatal mortality rate: The number of newborn deaths among those less than 3 months over the total number of live infants born during that year.

B. Cause specific mortality rate: The number of deaths that have occurred among those with a specific disease or disorder.

C. Case fatality rate: The number of deaths from a specific cause divided by the number of people in the population.

D. Proportionate mortality rate: The number of deaths attributable to a specific cause over the total number of deaths during a specific period of time.

71. Your patient is adversely affected with tetanus and they ask what kind of disease this is. What is your best response to this patient?

A. "You have a communicable disease."

B. "You have an infectious disease."

C. "You have a contagious disease."

D. "You have a non-preventable infection."

72. Quarantine can apply to:

A. Only those people who have become ill with a contagious disease

B. People who are ill with a serious and potentially fatal infectious disease

C. Buildings

D. Geographic areas regardless of risk

73. Which definition most accurately defines epidemiology?

A. The study of infections, their mode of transmission and prevention

B. The science of microorganisms and how they lead to infection

C. The study of health and illness patterns and determinants in populations

D. The assessment, planning, implementation and evaluation of infection control efforts.

74. The first three steps of epidemiological investigations and corrective action in correct sequential order are:

A. The definition of the problem or infectious situation, the description of the course or natural history of the event and the identification of points of control

B. The description of the course or natural history of the event, the definition of the problem or infectious situation and the generation of possible strategies that can stop and/or reverse the course of the event

C. The description of the course or natural history of the event, the generation of possible strategies that can stop and/or reverse the course of the event, the selection of strategies with the highest possibility of success and the design of strategic implementation.

D. The description of the problem or course of the event, the generation of possible strategies that can stop and/or reverse the course of the event, the selection of strategies with the highest possibility of success and the design of strategic implementation.

75. Which epidemiological model consists of the agent, host and environment?

A. The Web of Causation

B. The Wheel of Causation

C. The Determinants of Health

D. The Epidemiological Triad

76. Of all of the following, which is the most difficult to determine and scientifically substantiate?

A. Correlation

B. Causality

C. Multiple regression

D. Measures of central tendency

77. Which of the following is one of the components necessary to establish a cause and effect relationship?

A. Validity

B. Reliability

C. Consistency

D. Significance

78. Select the component of causality that is accurately paired with its description:

A. Consistency: The association can be observed repeatedly among different populations and at different times

B. Plausibility: The data can be feasibly collected in a longitudinal manner

C. Biological gradient: The explanation makes sense biologically

D. Temporality: The data collection is collected prospectively

79. As part of your performance improvement and quality assurance program you review your entire infection control program in terms of its completeness and accuracy. What are you studying as part of this review?

A. Outcomes

B. Processes

C. Structures

D. Administrative tools

80. After the review of your infection control program in terms of accuracy and completeness, you decide you want to study and explore the employee health program to determine that health assessments are done in a timely and efficient manner. What are you studying as part of this review?

A. Outcomes

B. Processes

C. Structures

D. Administrative tools

81. You have just completed a series of educational programs for clinical staff relating to the prevention of MRSA infections. You intend to look at the number of MRSA infections at the current time and then collect data about the number of MRSA infections six months after this educational series and, again, one year after the completion of the educational series. What kind of data are you collecting?

   A. Formative evaluation data

   B. Structure data

   C. Process data

   D. Outcomes data

82. The primary purpose of risk management activities, in contrast to quality improvement activities, is to:

   A. Decrease hospital acquired infections

   B. Decrease legal liability

   C. Increase JCAHO compliance

   D. Increase the quality of care

83. High inter-observer consistency over time is an indication of a measurement tool's:

   A. High reliability

   B. High validity

   C. Predictive ability

   D. High construct validity

84. After using a screening tool for the risks associated with pressure ulcers, you find that a high number of patients who were positive for risk did not develop any pressure ulcers. What aspect of this tool and its measurements should you be concerned about?

A. Its positive predictive value

B. Its poor predictive value

C. Its lack of validity

D. Its lack of timeliness

85. You will be doing a research study on the distribution of sexually transmitted diseases among adolescent ranging in age from 12 to 18 years of age. What type of research study will you be doing?

A. An analytic research study

B. An experimental research study

C. A quasi-experimental research study

D. A descriptive research study

86. Which research design uses only retrospective data?

A. A longitudinal study

B. A case control study

C. Prospective cohort studies

D. Experimental studies

87. Which design is used for qualitative research?

A. Meta-analysis design

B. Cross sectional design

C. Focus group design

D. Non experimental design

88. What type of statistics does the bell shape curve represent?

A. Multiple regression

B. Chi square

C. T test

D. Mode

89. The two major types of statistics are:

A. Qualitative and quantitative

B. Measures of variability and measures of central tendency

C. Inferential and experimental

D. Descriptive and inferential

90. What is the mean of this series? 12, 5, 8, 19, 17, 24, 5

A. 12

B. 12.8

C. 13

D. 13.8

91. What is the median of this series? 12, 5, 8, 19, 17, 24, 5

A. 5

B. 8

C. 12

D. 17

92. What is the mode of this series? 12, 5, 8, 19, 17, 24, 5

A. 5

B. 8

C. 12

D. 17

93. Which statistical method includes range, variance and standard deviation?

A. Inferential statistics

B. Measures of central tendency

C. Measures of variability

D. Deductive statistics

94. When the bell shaped curve has a longer tail on the left side than on the right, it is referred to as a:

A. Negative skew

B. Positive skew

C. Negative correlation

D. Positive correlation

95. The mean, median and mode are identical when there is a:

A. Correlation.

B. Skew.

C. Universal distribution.

D. Normal distribution.

96. What is the range of this series? 12, 5, 8, 19, 17, 24, 5

A. 5

B. 8

C. 12

D. 19

97. You have noticed that the number of postoperative infections has decreased when the number of people attending a preoperative educational program for patients increases. What type of correlation coefficient will be yielded when this data is analyzed?

A. A type I correlation coefficient

B. A type II correlation coefficient

C. A positive correlation coefficient

D. A negative correlation coefficient

98. Which of the following is not an inferential statistical method?

A. Standard deviation

B. Analysis of variance (ANOVA)

C. Analysis of covariance (ANCOVA)

D. Regression analysis

99. When does a type I statistical error occur?

A. When mathematical calculations occur during the initial stages of data analysis

B. When mathematical calculations are highly faulty and they nullify the results

C. When the null hypothesis is rejected and it should have been accepted

D. When the null hypothesis is accepted and it should have been rejected

100. Your hypothesis states that "The number of MRSA infections will decrease after visitors have learned the correct method of hand washing". What is the dependent variable?

A. A negative correlation hypothesis

B. A positive correlation hypothesis

C. The number of MRSA infections

D. The correct method of hand washing

101. Your hypothesis states that "The number of MRSA infections will decrease after visitors have learned the correct method of hand washing". What is the independent variable?

A. A negative correlation hypothesis

B. A positive correlation hypothesis

C. The number of MRSA infections

D. The correct method of hand washing

102. Your hypothesis states that "The number of MRSA infections will decrease after visitors have learned the correct method of hand washing". You find that there was no change in the number of infections after visitors learned about correct method of hand washing. You should report these findings as:

A. Failed

B. Insignificant

C. Accepting of the null hypothesis

D. Extraneous variables

103. Select the risk stratification technique that is accurately paired with its description.

A. Threshold modeling: Implementing inclusion data before sample selection

B. Clinical review: Implementing exclusion data before sample selection

C. Statistic modeling: Implementing inclusion data before sample selection

D. Variance review: Implementing exclusion data before sample selection

104. Which one of the following is one of the biggest challenges associated with determining post discharge surgical infections?

A. The lack of surgeon reporting

B. The lack of discharge notes

C. The lack of control over factors external to the healthcare facility

D. The lack of control over internal healthcare facility factors

105. You are using a patient satisfaction measurement tool that has several statements like the one below. Which measurement tool are you using?

"The infection control professional spoke to me in an understandable manner."				
1 Strongly Disagree	2 Disagree	3 Neither Agree nor Disagree	4 Agree	5 Strongly Agree

A. A Likert scale

B. A Guttman scale

C. A Multiple Choice scale

D. A Burke scale

106. Which scale collects data based on the premise that those who agree to one statement will agree to items of lower rank?

A. A Likert scale

B. A Guttman scale

C. A Rank scale

D. A Priority scale

107. Which type of questionnaire has the greatest response rate?

A. A mailed questionnaire

B. An e mailed questionnaire

C. A written questionnaire

D. A telephone questionnaire

108. Which statement about focus groups is accurate?

A. Focus groups generate quantitative data.

B. Questions and answers are highly structured.

C. Judgments about member responses prevent bias.

D. Groups are limited to six to ten members.

109. You are collecting observational data. You have informed your subjects that you will be observing their performance of wound care. What classification of observation is this?

A. No concealment with intervention

B. No concealment without intervention

C. Concealment with intervention

D. Concealment without intervention

110. When you state, "Tell me about your pain," you can expect:

A. An open-ended question response

B. An open-ended quantitative response

C. A close-ended question response

D. A close-ended quantitative response

111. Which form of data is most useful in terms of solving everyday practical problems?

A. Qualitative data

B. Inferential data

C. Deductive data

D. Critical incident data

112. Qualitative data is analyzed by:

A. Identifying themes and patterns

B. Using critical thinking

C. Using deductive reasoning

D. Socratic questioning

113. A research study states that p < .05. What does this mean?

A. There is < 95 % possibility that chance or accident has occurred.

B. There is < 5 % possibility that chance or accident has occurred.

C. There is < 95 % possibility that the findings are significant.

D. There is < 5 % possibility that the findings are significant.

114. Which statistic test indicates level of significance?

A. The standard deviation

B. The mean

C. The Chi square

D. Multiple regression

115. Which level of significance is the most rigorous?

A. $p < .01$

B. $p > .01$

C. $p < .95$

D. $p > .95$

116. Which agency collaborates with the CDC, state and local public health departments, the FDA and the Department of Agriculture to track all changes in the antimicrobial susceptibility of certain enteric bacteria, food animals and meats?

A. The United States Environmental Protection Agency

B. The United States Department of the Aging

C. The American Nurses Association

D. The National Antimicrobial Resistance Monitoring System for Enteric Bacteria

117. Which antibiotic resistant bacteria are classified as "serious" by the CDC?

A. Clostridium difficile

B. Vancomycin-resistant Enterococcus

C. Carbapenem-resistant Enterobacteriae (CRE)

D. Drug-resistant Neisseria gonorrhoeae

118. Which antibiotic resistant bacteria is classified as "concerning" by the CDC?

A. Carbapenem-resistant Enterobacteriae (CRE)

B. Drug-resistant Neisseria gonorrhoeae

C. Clindamycin-resistant Group B

D. Clostridium difficile

119. Which of the following is considered an internal performance benchmarking activity?

A. Comparing the infection control performances of members of your nursing staff and those of your neighboring facility

B. Comparing the infection control performances of members of the nursing and laboratory departments of your facility

C. A complete concurrent review of all the structures within your infection control and prevention department

D. A complete concurrent review of all the processes within your infection control and prevention department

120. A fishbone diagram is used to:

A. Display processes and decision points from the beginning to the end of the process

B. Display processes and functions and their interactions with other processes and functions

C. Factors that negatively impact on the process under study

D. Factors that impact on the process under study

121. Which graph, table or chart uses standard deviation calculations?

A. A histogram

B. A bar graph

C. A control chart

D. A Pareto chart

122. The force of facilitators must be stronger than the barriers to change, according to which theory or concept?

A. Havelock's Six Phases of Planned Change

B. Lewin's Forced Field Analysis

C. Roger's Innovation-Decision Process

D. Chaos Theory

123. Select the theorist and stage of change associated with an individual/group accepting and implementing desired change.

A. Rogers: Freezing

B. Rogers: Unfreezing

C. Lewin: Freezing

D. Lewin: Refreezing

124. Which theory states that a change agent provides the patient with knowledge and information about the benefits of change?

A. Havelock

B. Rogers

C. Orem

D. Lippitt

125. Which decision making step identifies important criteria?

A. Identifying the purpose

B. Establishing criteria

C. Ranking and weighing criteria

D. Exploring the alternatives in terms of established criteria

126. Which step of the decision making process involves 'what are the alternatives in the situation'?

A. Identifying the purpose

B. Establishing criteria

C. Ranking and weighing criteria

D. Exploring the alternatives in terms of established criteria

127. Which step of the decision making process involves 'the team observing the effects of the intervention'?

A. Exploring and forecasting risks that could result from the selected alternative

B. Evaluating the outcome

C. Implementation of the selected course of action

D. Ranking and weighing criteria

128. Which step of the decision making process involves 'what the risks are and what can be done to prevent or minimize the risk(s)'?

A. Exploring and forecasting risks that could result from the selected alternative

B. Evaluating the outcome

C. Implementation of the selected course of action

D. Ranking and weighing criteria

129. Match the CDC's type of "case" with its correct description.

A. Confirmed case: A case that is confirmed with at least one laboratory method listed in the definition of the specific case.

B. Clinically compatible case: A case with a collection of symptoms associated with a disease

C. Laboratory confirmed case: A case that is considered probable for reporting purposes.

D. Suspected case: A case where laboratory results are positive but not included in the laboratory Criteria for Diagnosis.

130. There are times when more than one screening instrument is used for the same disease or infection. What type of screening is this?

A. Stratified screening

B. High risk screening

C. Concurrent screening

D. Multiphasic screening

131. What term is used to describe the radiation dose required to inactivate 90% of the test microorganism under stated exposure conditions?

A. Bioburden

B. D value

C. Bacterial count

D. Bio-percent

132. **Which device consists of a standardized, viable population of microorganisms known to be resistant to the sterilization process?**

A. A chemical indicator

B. A sterilization indicator

C. A biologic indicator

D. A mechanical indicator

133. **One of the goals of the central supply area is to eradicate all extraneous material from medical items. The process is referred to as:**

A. Disinfection

B. Partial disinfection

C. Cleaning

D. Sterilization

134. **Which method tests sterilization?**

A. Rideal Walker Method

B. Chick Martin test

C. Koch's method

D. Mechanical indicator

135. What is a class II recall?

A. The item can cause highly serious adverse health consequences

B. The item can cause irreversible health consequences

C. The item is not likely to lead to any health consequences

D. The item can cause temporary and reversible consequences

136. Select the bioterrorism agent accurately paired with its category.

A. Category A: Q fever

B. Category B: Smallpox

C. Category C: Nipah virus

D. Category D: Psittacosis

137. Which bioterrorism agent is not transmissible without direct contact?

A. Tularemia

B. Anthrax

C. Smallpox

D. Bubonic plague

138. Your patient is diagnosed with Bang's fever. Which is the most likely way that they have been infected?

A. With contaminated meat

B. With an aerosol

C. With a droplet

D. By a flea bite

139. Which infection has Horder's spots as a symptom?

A. Brucellosis

B. Q Fever

C. Psittacosis

D. Ricin

140. Which fact about leadership is accurate?

A. Leaders are born with the characteristics of leadership

B. Staff at the highest level of the organization are the only leaders

C. Leadership is inherent and can't be learned

D. Staff at the lowest level of the organization can be leaders

141. Which theory of leadership states that leaders respond with certain behaviors according to the particular situation?

A. The Michigan Leadership Studies Managerial Grid

B. The Charismatic Theory

C. The Great Man Theory

D. The Contingency Theory

142. Which of the following theorists are credited with the Six Emotional Leadership Styles?

A. Hersey and Blanchard

B. Goleman, Boyatzis and McKee

C. Flamholtz and Randle

D. Likert and Guttman

143. Select the type of leadership that is accurately paired with Likert's description of it:

A. Exploitative Authoritative: Leaders motivate others with common goals and concrete tasks. punishments, fear and threats.

B. Consultative: This style is the most effective and satisfying because there is full participation in decision making and a reward system is in place.

C. Participative: This style facilitates higher levels of motivation, increased job satisfaction and greater productivity than the benevolent authoritative and authoritative styles of leadership.

D. Benevolent Authoritative: This style has less punishment and more rewards than the exploitive authoritative style of leadership.

144. Your department director gives team members a great amount of freedom and autonomy in terms of what, how and when tasks are done, but is readily available to provide guidance and support when needed. What type of leadership style is this director employing?

A. Democratic leadership

B. Participative leadership

C. Laissez faire leadership

D. Autocratic leadership

145. Which of the following are some of the Six Leadership Styles of Goleman, Boyatzis and McKee?

A. Affiliative, commanding and pacesetting

B. Consultative, directive and democratic

C. Democratic, participative and laissez faire

D. Primary, secondary and tertiary

146. The leadership model of Flamholtz and Randle states that leaders:

A. Should use a style that is congruent with the team member's level of competency.

B. Have four leadership tasks and all must be incorporated into all interactions.

C. Have three leadership tasks and all must be incorporated into all interactions.

D. Should use a style that is the most comfortable for the leader and their skills.

147. The acceptance of a caring touch is an example of what?

A. A universal need

B. A universal preference

C. A cultural communication variable

D. A cultural religious variable

148. Which statement about personal spaces is accurate?

A. Personal spaces vary according to religion

B. Personal spaces vary among cultures

C. Personal spaces are specifically defined for all cultures

D. Personal spaces lack scientific merit

149. Select the personal space that is paired with its correct definition in terms of distance.

A. The Intimate Zone: 6 inches to 1 foot of distance from the body.

B. The Personal Zone: From 1 ½ feet to 6 feet in distance.

C. The Social Zone: 6 feet to 12 feet.

D. The Public Zone: Over 12 feet from the person.

150. "The American Red Cross prevents and alleviates human suffering in the face of emergencies by mobilizing the power of volunteers and the generosity of donors" is an example of what?

A. A mission statement

B. A value statement

C. A principle statement

D. An objectives statement

ANSWER KEY

1. d	39. c	77. c	115. a
2. b	40. c	78. a	116. d
3. c	41. b	79. c	117. b
4. d	42. b	80. b	118. c
5. b	43. c	81. d	119. a
6. a	44. d	82. b	120. d
7. a	45. c	83. a	121. c
8. c	46. c	84. b	122. b
9. a	47. a	85. d	123. d
10. c	48. c	86. b	124. b
11. d	49. b	87. c	125. c
12. d	50. a	88. d	126. d
13. a	51. b	89. d	127. c
14. b	52. a	90. b	128. a
15. a	53. c	91. c	129. b
16. c	54. b	92. b	130. d
17. d	55. c	93. c	131. b
18. c	56. b	94. a	132. c
19. a	57. a	95. d	133. c
20. a	58. c	96. d	134. d
21. b	59. a	97. d	135. d
22. c	60. b	98. a	136. c
23. d	61. a	99. c	137. b
24. d	62. d	100. c	138. a
25. c	63. a	101. d	139. c
26. c	64. b	102. c	140. d
27. a	65. c	103. a	141. d
28. d	66. b	104. c	142. b
29. c	67. c	105. a	143. d
30. c	68. d	106. b	144. d
31. d	69. b	107. d	145. a
32. b	70. d	108. d	146. a
33. c	71. b	109. b	147. c
34. b	72. c	110. a	148. b
35. d	73. c	111. d	149. d
36. d	74. a	112. a	150. a
37. b	75. d	113. b	
38. d	76. b	114. c	

CBIC Essential Test Tips DVD from Trivium Test Prep!

Dear Customer,

Thank you for purchasing from Trivium Test Prep! We're honored to help you prepare for your CBIC.

To show our appreciation, we're offering a **FREE *CBIC Essential Test Tips* DVD by Trivium Test Prep**. Our DVD includes 35 test preparation strategies that will make you successful on the CBIC. All we ask is that you email us your feedback and describe your experience with our product. Amazing, awful, or just so-so: we want to hear what you have to say!

To receive your **FREE *CBIC Essential Test Tips* DVD**, please email us at 5star@triviumtestprep.com. Include "Free 5 Star" in the subject line and the following information in your email:

1. The title of the product you purchased.
2. Your rating from 1 – 5 (with 5 being the best).
3. Your feedback about the product, including how our materials helped you meet your goals and ways in which we can improve our products.
4. Your full name and shipping address so we can send your FREE "#$"! %&&)*+,!-' &)!-*.&DVD.

If you have any questions or concerns please feel free to contact us directly at 5star@triviumtestprep.com. Thank you!

- Trivium Test Prep Team

CPSIA information can be obtained
at www.ICGtesting.com
Printed in the USA
LVHW052257290720
661911LV00019B/1743